# Certified Nurse Educator (CNE) Review Manual

**Ruth A. Wittmann-Price, PhD, RN, CNS, CNE,** is an Assistant Professor at Drexel University College of Nursing and Health Professions. She received her AAS and BSN from Felician College in Lodi, New Jersey, in 1978 and 1981, respectively. She received her MS from Columbia University in New York City in 1983 as a perinatal CNS. She has worked as a mother-baby nurse for over 30 years. In 2006 she completed her PhD at Widener University and was awarded the Dean's Award for Excellence in Scholarship. She has been teaching nursing for over 10 years and sat for the first CNE examination in Baltimore in 2005. She was the recipient of the 2008 Nursing Spectrum Regional Award for excellence in teaching. She has coedited a nursing education book *Nursing Education: Foundations of Practice Excellence,* which won the 2008 AJN book of the year award in the category for teaching. Dr. Wittmann-Price's research areas include women's health decisions and she has published on her theory on emancipated decision making. Other research interests include developmental care of the preterm infant.

**Maryann Godshall, MSN, RN, CCRN, CPN,** is an Assistant Professor at DeSales University in the Department of Nursing and Health. She received her BSN from Allentown College of St. Francis DeSales and her MSN from DeSales University. She has a post-master's degree in Nursing Education from Duquesne University and is a PhD candidate at Duquesne University. She has been teaching for 9 years and her expertise is in pediatrics. She holds a certification in both pediatrics and pediatric critical care. Her current research interest is with pediatric burn patients. She has published several articles and most recently a chapter in *Disaster Nursing* and *Maternal Child Nursing Across the Lifespan.* Her accomplishments include the 2008 Nightingale Award of Pennsylvania Nursing Scholarship.

# Certified Nurse Educator (CNE) Review Manual

Ruth A. Wittmann-Price, PhD, RN, CNS, CNE
Maryann Godshall, MSN, RN, CCRN, CPN
Editors

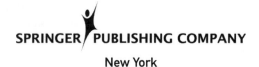

SPRINGER PUBLISHING COMPANY

New York

Springer Publishing Company, LLC
11 West 42nd Street
New York, NY 10036
www.springerpub.com

*Acquisitions Editor: Margaret Zuccarini*

*Project Manager: Mark Frazier*

*Cover Designer: David Levy*

*Composition: Apex CoVantage, LLC*

Ebook ISBN: 978-0826-10506-6

09  10  11  12  13 / 5  4  3  2

**Library of Congress Cataloging-in-Publication Data**

Wittmann-Price, Ruth A.
  Certified nurse educator (CNE) review manual / Ruth A. Wittmann-Price and Maryann Godshall.
     p. cm.
  Includes bibliographical references and index.
  ISBN 978-0-8261-0505-9 (alk. paper)
  1. Nursing schools—Faculty—Certification—Study guides.  2. Nursing—Practice—Examinations, questions, etc.  3. Nursing schools—Faculty—Vocational guidance.  4. Nursing—Study and teaching.  I. Godshall, Maryann. II. Title.
  RT90.W58 2009
  610.73076—dc22                                                          2009014205

Printed in the United States of America by Hamilton Printing.

# Contents

**Chapter 9** *Functioning Effectively Within the Institutional Environment and Academic Community* . . . . . . . . . . . . . . . . . . . . 213
**Mary Ellen Smith Glasgow**

# Contributors

**Diane M. Billings, EdD, RN, FAAN**
Chancellor's Professor Emeritus
Indiana University School of Nursing
Indianapolis, IN

**Fran Cornelius, PhD, RN-BC, CNE**
Associate Clinical Professor and Coordinator of Informatics Projects
Drexel University
College of Nursing & Health Professions
Philadelphia, PA

**Rosemary Fliszar, PhD, RN, CNE**
Assistant Professor
Kutztown University
Kutztown, PA

**Mary Gallagher-Gordon, MSN, RN, CNE**
Assistant Professor
Drexel University
College of Nursing & Health Professions
Philadelphia, PA

**Mary Ellen Smith Glasgow, PhD, RN, CS**
Associate Professor & Associate Dean for Undergraduate Programs,
MSN Programs & Continuing Nursing Education
Drexel University
College of Nursing & Health Professions
Philadelphia, PA

**Marylou K. McHugh, EdD, RN, CNE**
Associate Professor
Drexel University
College of Nursing & Health Professions
Philadelphia, PA

**Brenda Reap Thompson, MSN, RN, CNE**
Clinical Assistant Professor and Director of NCLEX Education
for Continuing Nursing Education
Drexel University
College of Nursing & Health Professions
Philadelphia, PA

**Linda Wilson, PhD, RN, CPAN, CAPA, BC, CNE**
Assistant Professor
Drexel University
College of Nursing & Health Professions
Philadelphia, PA

# Foreword

One of the effects of the nursing faculty shortage has been a heightened awareness of the important role of educators in schools of nursing and clinical settings. This awareness has extended beyond nursing education to the general public, with news reports informing readers about qualified applicants to nursing programs being turned away because of the lack of faculty to teach them. The current faculty shortage has occurred for a number of reasons, including fewer graduate students preparing for educator roles to replace the number of faculty who are retiring, difficulties in recruiting clinicians and administrators to teach in schools of nursing because of the lower salaries of faculty compared with healthcare settings, and until recently, limited numbers of programs to prepare nurse educators. The awareness of the need for nurse educators, combined with the reality of decreasing numbers of faculty, has led to the growth of Master's, Doctoral (both PhD and DNP), and certificate programs to prepare nurse educators and the development of strategies such as scholarships and loans to encourage graduate students to consider a career in nursing education (Oermann, 2005). However, the current economic recession threatens the gain nursing has made in recent years to increase the number of educators.

Accompanying these trends is the recognition that nursing education has a body of knowledge to be learned, and that there are core competencies to be developed for the expert teaching of nursing. Nurse educators need an understanding of learning concepts and theories, principles of curriculum development and course planning, and their roles and responsibilities in those areas. Across all settings in which students learn, nurse educators must be skilled in planning instruction for students with varying learning needs and abilities, selecting appropriate teaching methods, presenting information effectively to small and large groups of learners, integrating active learning methods within classes and courses, and demonstrating evidence-based clinical teaching skills. Today's faculty needs a breadth of knowledge and competencies because their roles also may include teaching distance education courses, in simulation laboratories, and with innovative instructional methods and technologies.

Educators not only teach, they also are responsible for assessing and evaluating students' learning outcomes and clinical competencies. Assessment is the collection of information about student learning and performance, and provides a basis for identifying learning needs and deciding on instructional activities to promote further learning. Assessment also helps educators to confirm that students have met the desired outcomes and developed necessary clinical competencies. Evaluation is the process of making judgments about those outcomes and competencies, based on the assessment data (Broadfoot, 2007; Oermann & Gaberson, 2009).

Nurse educators function within institutions, and, as such, need to understand the environment in which they teach and its effects on their roles and responsibilities. The mission and goals of the setting influence the educator's role. Differences across schools of nursing in tenure and promotion requirements, criteria for clinical and tenure tracks for nursing faculty, and expectations of faculty are striking. To be successful, the teacher needs to understand those requirements and expectations.

Across all settings, the nurse educator is a leader and change agent, participating in efforts to improve nursing education, developing educational innovations, and gaining leadership skills. Once prepared as a nurse educator, one's own learning and professional development continues. Educators need to expand their own knowledge and skills and be committed to participating in career development activities. As faculty foster the value of lifelong learning among students, so too are faculty lifelong learners.

Decisions made about educational practices should be based on sound evidence, generated through research studies that are of high quality. Much of the current research in nursing education, though, is done with small samples, in one setting, and with questionable tools. We cannot identify best practices in nursing education without high quality research studies. In some areas of nursing education, however, there is evidence to guide teaching, but how many educators routinely check the literature as a basis for their educational decisions? The role of nurse educator as scholar not only includes conducting research and disseminating findings but also approaching one's teaching by questioning current practices and searching for evidence to answer those questions (Oermann, 2009).

Many health fields offer certifications to acknowledge expertise in a specialty area of practice or role, and there is evidence to support positive outcomes of certifications (Wade, 2009). Similar to certifications in clinical specialties, certification in nursing education is a means for teachers to demonstrate their knowledge about nursing education and expertise in the educator role. The National League for Nursing offers certification in nursing education through its Certified Nurse Educator (CNE®) examination. That examination assesses the teacher's knowledge about learning, curriculum development, teaching methods, assessment and evaluation, academic institutions, quality improvement as a nurse educator, and scholarship in nursing education. It serves as a means of documenting advanced knowledge, expertise, and competencies in the role of nurse educator.

This book was developed as a resource for nurse educators to prepare themselves to take *and pass* the CNE examination. It includes valuable information for this purpose and also serves as a review of important principles for effective teaching in nursing. The book describes the concepts and principles that define nursing education, describes the core competencies of nurse educators, and provides a perspective of expert teaching in nursing. This book is a valuable resource for nurse educators in preparing for the CNE examination and for aspiring teachers in nursing.

*Marilyn H. Oermann, PhD, RN, FAAN, ANEF*
*Professor and Division Chair, School of Nursing*
*University of North Carolina at Chapel Hill*
*Chapel Hill, North Carolina*

# References

Broadfoot, P. (2007). *An introduction to assessment.* New York: Continuum.

Oermann, M. H. (2005). Post-master's certificate in nursing education: Strategy for preparing nursing faculty. *International Journal of Nursing Education Scholarship, 2*(1), art. 8. Retrieved March 24, 2009, from http://www.bepress.com/ijnes/vol2/iss1/art8/

Oermann, M. H. (2009). Evidence-based programs and teaching/evaluation methods: Needed achieve excellence in nursing education. In M. Adams & T. Valiga (Eds.), *Achieving Excellence in Nursing Education.* New York: National League for Nursing.

Oermann, M. H., & Gaberson, K. (2009). *Evaluation and testing in nursing education* (3rd ed.). New York: Springer Publishing.

Wade, C. H. (2009). Perceived effects of specialty nurse certification: A review of the literature. *AORN Journal, 89,* 183–192.

# Preface

This book was created to assist in the advancement of the *nurse educator* role that is distinct from other advanced nursing roles. Most nurse educators would probably agree that teaching in nursing is a rewarding professional career. Witnessing a student or colleague become excited by the discovery, realization or mastery of new information, techniques, or skills is extremely gratifying. The classroom, clinical, and staff development realms all fall within the expertise of the nurse educator. These realms are parts of larger systems that nurse educators navigate successfully to accomplish their goal of knowledge development. In any one classroom or clinical setting, facilitating the education of others is not only a rewarding experience but also a role that greatly impacts the future of healthcare.

In the past, nurse educators had no formal education to prepare them to teach, they were simply content experts who learned the educational pedagogy by trial and error. Now, nursing education is recognized as a specialty with a distinct body of knowledge. Like nursing, it is an applied science. This book will highlight areas outlined by our National League of Nursing (NLN) as essential knowledge needed for the nurse educator to excel in the field and pass the Certified Nurse Educator® (CNE) exam.

The competencies for nurse educators from the NLN Web site are listed at the beginning of each chapter. Competency is best defined by *WordNet*® *3.0.* (n.d.) as "the quality of being adequately or well qualified physically and intellectually." Competence can be viewed as a minimal skill set or level that must be achieved to pass. Excellence means "possessing good qualities in high degree" (*WordNet*® *3.0,* n.d.). The CNE publicly confers that distinction upon nurse educators.

Nursing leaders developed the CNE to recognize and capture excellence in nursing education. Since the first exam was offered to 174 candidates as a pencil and paper test in Baltimore, Maryland, on September 28, 2005, over 1,400 nurse educators have passed the exam (National League of Nursing, 2009). Those nurse educators proudly display the CNE initials after their names.

To prepare nurse educators for the certification exam, the NLN provides an extensive bibliography, preparation course, and practice tests that may be accessed from their informative Web site (http://www.nln.org/facultycertification/index.htm). These resources are invaluable for nurse educators preparing to take the CNE examination. This book is an adjunct to those resources and has been written because many nurse educators have asked us how we prepared for the first exam in 2005.

This book should been seen as a supplement to the materials already available from the NLN. It was developed independently from the NLN in order to further assist nurse educators in gaining confidence about taking the exam. The book is modeled after the NLN published test plan. Many of the areas in the test plan overlap, therefore you may find topics in this book that have content in two places but they will be cross-referenced. This is also the nature of nursing education; it is an interwoven realm of content, context, and process wherein each area affects another. We hope this book captures the essence of information nurse educators need to move to a recognized level of excellence. We have included additional references and teaching gems for those who would like further explanation and exploration of topics, and we encourage you to use these. We have searched out evidence to support our content and have inserted research when applicable into each chapter. Further, we have included clearly designated, evidence-based education boxes to help hone your focus on the evidence and discoveries of fellow educators. You will also find case studies at the end of each chapter to promote critical thinking and sample test questions that may be similar to those found on the CNE exam.

Chapter 1 covers some of the specifics of the CNE exam and reviews test taking skills.

Chapter 2 reviews how a nurse educator facilitates learning by assessing the learning needs and skills of his or her students. It also reviews learner outcomes and teaching strategies and discusses how to adapt them to the students' own experiences. This is important for an educator to assess in order to develop an appropriate teaching plan. Another area discussed in the chapter is how the nurse educator serves as a role model for the students and assists them in becoming motivated and enthusiastic about learning.

Chapter 3 is devoted to socialization skills needed by students and speaks to the ever-increasing diversity in culture and styles that affects nursing education. Another important aspect of Chapter 3 is its examination of resources for students who are at risk for any number of reasons that may affect them perceptually, cognitively, physically, or culturally. Incivility is also addressed in relation to today's teaching environment.

Chapter 4 discusses evaluation strategies used by nurse educators and how they balance the aspects of admission, progression, and retention to ensure good program outcomes. Effective evaluation tools are extremely important in the process of student success and public safety.

Chapter 5 addresses the larger institutional considerations of curriculum design and evaluation. The chapter analyzes how courses are developed within a curriculum and how a curriculum flows. The chapter also discusses how the curriculum interfaces with the mission of the institution and the community.

Chapter 6 highlights professional development for nurse educators and how educators navigate their role to become mentors to the next generation of nurse educators. Learning for educators is life-long and has increased in intensity exponentially with the accelerating advancements in information and technology. This chapter provides nurse educators with ideas on how to keep abreast of developments and advancements in the educational field.

Chapter 7 speaks to the nurse educator's role as a leader who interfaces with the larger community of academics and administrators. This chapter examines nursing's place in the larger systems and how nurse educators can effect change in those systems.

Chapter 8 dissects the scholarship needed for nurse educators to stay on top of their game. "Publish or perish" is a phenomenon known to academics and is also applicable to nurse educators in an academic setting. This chapter discusses types of scholarship and professional plans to enable nurse educators to become proficient at publishing. The chapter also emphasizes the importance of disseminating nursing knowledge.

Chapter 9 discusses interdisciplinary collaboration within institutions for nurse educators. Nursing has a longer history of being taught in stand-alone schools than it does as part of a larger educational community. Nurse educators have assimilated into the larger community as experts in a field that has the unique position of being both clinical and didactic, and the professionalism that we bring to the larger academic community has enhanced the standings of many institutions and colleges. Nursing is a visible professional entity that collaborates and contributes to the overall mission of the institution and society.

We have developed this book to assist you in your preparation for the CNE exam, but know that it only glazes each area that may be evaluated. Our hope is that it will serve you as another tool to reach your goal of recognized excellence. We applaud your efforts as colleagues in the quest to educate the next generation of nurses, and thank you for your efforts to recognize excellence in our field. We also want to encourage you to provide feedback on our Web site so that we may incorporate your feedback into the next edition of this book.

*Ruth A. Wittmann-Price, PhD, RN, CNS, CNE*
*Maryann Godshall, MSN, RN, CCRN, CPN*

## References

National League of Nursing. (2009). Certification for Educators. Retrieved December 29, 2008, from http://www.nln.org/facultycertification/index.htm

*WordNet® 3.0.* (n.d.). Competency. Retrieved July 4, 2008, from http://dictionary.reference.com/browse/competency

# Acknowledgments

Thank you to all of my students over the years who have taught me and continue to teach me a tremendous amount about nursing, life, and humility, and to Angela Pasco, director of the Schuylkill Health School of Nursing, my first mentor in nursing education.

*Ruth A. Wittmann-Price*

Thank you to the nursing students who have allowed me to grow as an educator and for sharing some of the most cherished moments I have ever experienced while touching the lives of children. May we both never stop learning. I would also like to thank Ruth Wittmann-Price for being my mentor, and motivator, and for her never ending support of my work.

*Maryann Godshall*

Thank you to the National League for Nursing for allowing us to use specific CNE Core Competencies, from *The Scope of Practice for Academic Nurse Educators* (2005), as the focal points of individual chapters.

Thank you to Doug Graup for the artwork.

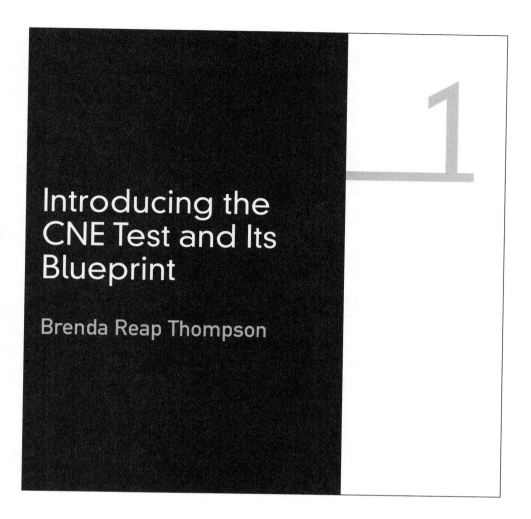

# Introducing the CNE Test and Its Blueprint

Brenda Reap Thompson

*Nursing is an art: and if it is to be made an art, it requires an exclusive devotion as hard a preparation, as any painter's or sculptor's work; for what is the having to do with dead canvas or dead marble, compared with having to do with the living body, the temple of God's spirit? It is one of the Fine Arts: I had almost said, the finest of Fine Arts.*

—Florence Nightingale

## Learning Outcomes

- Identify the processes to best prepare for the CNE exam.
- Utilize the tips for success to promote understanding and learning of key concepts.
- Integrate the CNE competencies with your current academic experience.
- Improve comprehension by eliminating anxiety related to test taking.

## Introduction

Nurse educators' certification comes at a time in history when nursing is actively recruiting advanced, practiced nurses into the educational realm. This recruitment process is imperative to offset the current and impending nursing shortage taking place in the United States today. The shortage is actually twofold: there is a lack of nurses and there is a lack of nurse educators. The U.S. Bureau of Labor Statistics (2007) predicts that there will be a shortage of over 500,000 nurses by the year 2016. The shortage of bedside nurses is, in part, being created by the United States' aging demographics related to the maturing baby boomers, a group sporting more chronic illnesses than any prior generation. Second, the American Academy of Colleges of Nursing (AACN) reports that, ironically, nursing schools turned away 40,285 qualified applicants from baccalaureate and graduate nursing programs in 2007 due to inadequate numbers of faculty, clinical sites, classroom space, clinical preceptors, and budget constraints (American Academy of Colleges of Nursing, 2009).

A 50% increase in nursing graduates by 2020 is needed to meet the United States' demand for nurses. A substantial increase in student nurses is only one factor that summons the urgency for certified nursing faculty. Another contributing factor adding to the faculty shortage is the demographics of the current teaching faculty. The average age of a Master's prepared faculty member is 49, while the average age of those holding Doctorate degrees is 53. The average age of retirement for nursing faculty is 62.5 years. A projected peak retirement period for faculty in this country is estimated to begin in the year 2010 (Yordy, 2006).

Many colleges and schools of nursing are recruiting expert nurse clinicians and advanced practice RNs to assist in filling their vacant academic and clinical faculty roles. This recruitment process has been fostered by state and foundational funds to supplement nurse educator programs on the Masters and Doctoral levels.

The role development that many nurse educators go through involves a transformation from an *expert* clinician to a *novice* educator. Nursing literature provides ample documentation to demonstrate that being an expert clinician does not provide an educator with the skill set he or she needs to become a successful teacher. Through additional studies that lead to certification in nursing education, expert clinicians can become comfortable in their new role as nurse educators and build their new practice, preparing the next generation of nurses, on solid teaching and learning principles.

Neese (2003) described this transformation from novice to expert in nursing education nicely by describing her stages based on Meizrow's (1991) adult learning concepts and Cranton's (2002) seven facets of transformational learning. These stages, as described by Neese, are a helpful framework for the intense learning that must take place to become comfortable in the role of an educator. These stages include:

- An activating event, usually a cumulative point in time when a nurse decides to leave clinical practice to pursue an educator role.
- Articulating assumptions is a process of self-reflection about "the baggage" one assumes about a process prior to embarking on it.

- Critical reflection challenging beliefs and *unlearning* (or, eliminating preexisting knowledge that may actually be a deterrent to new ideas).
- Opening oneself to alternative views and engaging in discourse.
- Revising one's original assumptions.
- Acting on revisions to help meet one's goal of becoming an educator.

Indeed, nurse educators with years of experience can validate their expertise and knowledge by certification. These educators are an invaluable resource to the current system and certified educators are sorely needed as mentors, role models, and visionaries to assist future nursing educators. Educators who complete the core competencies of a Certified Nurse Educator are needed to move the profession forward. The following list outlines just a few ways in which that progression will manifest itself:

- Mentors may assist new faculty with preparation for teaching, the development of test questions, grading, and decision-making.
- Versatile education styles are necessary for providing quality education to diverse populations.
- The role of an educator expands beyond the discipline of teaching and includes scholarship and service.

## Reaching for Academic Excellence

Academic excellence often is encouraged through an atmosphere that influences educators to challenge themselves to reach beyond their normal expectations. Faculty who support an atmosphere of excellence can thrive and their success will raise the bar and academic standards for the whole discipline.

- In many instances, high standards will eventually become the norm.
- Academic leadership standards, whether high or low, will trickle-down to affect the faculty as a whole.
- Preparing competent nurse educators should result in preparing competent students.

Your decision to take the CNE certification examination is a challenging experience which will allow you to test your competence as a nurse educator.

- Table 1.1 presents the content categories contained within the test blueprint and the percentage of each category in the National League for Nursing (NLN) (National League for Nursing [NLN], 2009a) Certified Nurse Educator (CNE) Examination.
- The following chapters in this CNE Review Manual present an in-depth explanation for each of the content areas that appear on the CNE Examination.

| Table 1.1 | Content of the CNE® Examination | |
|---|---|---|
| **Content** | | **Percentage of the Examination** |
| 1. | Facilitate learning | 25% |
| 2. | Facilitate learner development and socialization | 11% |
| 3. | Use assessment and evaluation strategies | 15% |
| 4. | Participate in curriculum design and evaluation of program outcomes | 19% |
| 5. | Pursue continuous quality improvement in the academic nurse educator role | 12% |
| 6. | Engage in scholarship, service, and leadership | |
| | A. Function as a change agent and leader | 8% |
| | B. Engage in scholarship of teaching | 5% |
| | C. Function effectively within the institutional environment and the academic community | 5% |

From *The scope of practice for academic nurse educators,* National League for Nursing (NLN), 2005, New York: National League for Nursing. Reprinted with Permission.

## Preparing for the CNE Examination

### Setting up a Study Schedule

When you create a study schedule, begin prioritizing the order in which you study the content by using the CNE Blueprint, as outlined in Table 1.1. Create a chart and divide your total studying time into eight sections and break up the total studying time into the percentages that correlate with the content percentage. The highest percentages of content covered in the examination are as follows (by category):

- Category 1: Facilitate Learning (25%) (Chapter 2)
- Category 4: Participate in Curriculum Design and Evaluation of Program Outcomes (19%) (Chapter 5)

The next-highest percentages of content covered in the examination are:

- Category 3: Use Assessment Strategies (15%) (Chapter 4)
- Category 5: Pursue Continuous Quality Improvement in the Academic Nurse Educator Role (12%) (Chapter 6)
- Category 2: Facilitate Learner Development and Socialization (11%) (Chapter 3)
- Category 6a: Function as a Change Agent and Leader (8%) (Chapter 7)

▪ Category 6b: Engage in Scholarship of Teaching (5%) (Chapter 8)
▪ Category 6c: Function Effectively within the Institutional Environment and the Academic Community (5%) (Chapter 9)

Employing the above strategy will help ensure that you will have time to review the categories that represent the highest percentage of questions on the CNE examination.

## Incorporating Key Topics Into Your Review for the CNE Examination

▪ Key topics for inclusion in your review include those in Exhibit 1.1.

| Exhibit 1.1 | Key Topics for Inclusion in Review |
|---|---|

| | |
|---|---|
| Teaching Styles—authoritarian, Socratic, heuristic, behavioral | Teaching—learning process |
| Active learning | Cooperative learning |
| Cooperative testing | Planning clinical learning experiences |
| Critical thinking activities—classroom and clinical | Characteristics of learners (cultural, traditional, nontraditional, educationally disadvantaged) |
| Domains—cognitive, psychomotor, affective | Promotion of professional responsibility—self-assessment, peer review |
| Graduation and retention rates | Academic appeals process |
| Bloom's Taxonomy | Test blueprint |
| Norm and criterion reference | Formative and summative evaluation |
| Test validity | Test reliability |
| Item discrimination ratio | Point biserial |
| Item difficulty | Program Standards—federal laws, state regulations, Professional Accreditation—the Commission on Collegiate Nursing Education (CCNE) and The National League for Nursing Accrediting Commission (NLNAC) |
| Credentialing—American Association of Colleges of Nursing (AACN) | Curriculum—mission statement, conceptual framework, level objectives, behavioral objectives, evaluation of learning outcomes (clinical and theoretical) |
| Curriculum evaluation—internal and external | Family Educational Rights and Privacy Act (FERPA)/Buckley Amendment |
| Audio conferencing | Video streaming |
| Synchronous and asynchronous methods of instruction | Types of leadership |
| Scholarship of discovery | Scholarship of teaching |
| Scholarship of practice (application) | Scholarship of integration |

## Planning and Registering for the CNE Examination

### Using the NLN Web Site to Establish Your Eligibility

Verify that you meet the eligibility requirements to take the exam. These requirements are listed on the NLN Web site.

- From the NLN Web site: http://www.nln.org/facultycertification/information/sae.htm. Click on *Certification for Nurse Educators*

Print the following materials from the Web site:

- Certified Nurse Educator (CNE) Candidate Handbook (NLN, 2009b)
- Detailed Test Blueprint
- List of Recommended References

Order the following materials from the Web site:

- The Scope of Practice for Academic Nurse Educators—there is an additional fee for this resource.
- Self-Assessment Examination (SAE)—this 65-item practice examination has multiple-choice questions in each category. The test can be taken multiple times over 60 days with available rationales. The score report is calculated in each of the six categories, so it can be used to focus studies within specific areas. (Note: there is a fee for this optional practice test).

Register to take the CNE Examination:

- Registration deadlines can be found on the Web site, so make sure you register in advance because you will need this confirmation to schedule your test.
- Click on the link to find the testing center nearest you.
- Current fees are available on the NLN Web site.
- Inquire from your faculty administrator if the test fee is reimbursable.

## Nuts and Bolts of the CNE Examination

### Become Familiar With the CNE Examination

- The examination has 150 items; 130 are operational and 20 are pretest items that do not count toward the score.
- Three hours are allotted to complete the examination, which includes a short tutorial.
- This allows approximately 1.2 minutes for each question.
- Avoid rapid guessing on the examination.

- Read questions carefully and answer items at a consistent pace.
- You can use your mouse to highlight important words in the question to improve your focus.

### Examination Items Requiring Additional Time

- Information about student grades that require math calculations
- Information about test item analysis that require a comparison of data

### Become Familiar With Electronic Testing Advantages

- If you are unsure of an answer, you can bookmark the question and return to it when you have completed the remainder of the examination.
- Use the arrows that allow you to page forward or backward during the examination if you want to change an answer; however, as educators we are aware that the first choice is usually correct.

## Tips for Success

### Incorporate Strategies to Ease the Fear of Test Anxiety

It is normal for a nurse educator to feel anxious about taking the CNE examination.

- As nurses, we know that anxiety is a natural response to the new challenges in our lives.
- Some anxiety will produce a heightened awareness and may improve test taking, while anxiety that is uncontrolled will impede the ability to think critically.
- Everyone who takes tests experiences anxiety; however, recognizing and controlling anxiety is the important key.

Some strategies that can be used to ease test anxiety include:

1. Reducing anxiety related to time constraints.
   - Schedule the examination when you have a semester that is less stressful.
   - Start a study group with other faculty and plan to meet once a week for two hours.
     - Use the detailed test plan to divide assignments.
     - Each faculty member can complete an assignment and share notes with the group.

■ Faculty members can also share the sources of information recommended by the NLN.

2. Reducing anxiety related to lack of recent experience in test taking.

   ■ After reviewing the content for the examination, complete as many test questions as possible, including the practice examination from NLN.
   ■ Self-evaluation will assist you in refocusing on specific content.
   ■ Practice will increase your confidence.

3. Reducing anxiety related to previous experience with testing difficulty.

   ■ Stop negative thoughts that begin with "what if."
   ■ Strategies such as positive self talk, daily exercise, yoga, and meditation have all been proven to decrease anxiety.
   ■ Practice these strategies on a regular basis so that decreasing anxiety becomes easy to achieve.

## Utilize Learning Strategies

### Remember by Comparison

An example of remembering by comparison is determining what information is the same and what is different among a variety of categories of information. This learning strategy focuses on the differences. An example of this learning strategy is illustrated here:

There are four types of scholarship. *All types of scholarship are peer reviewed and include research and grant awards. So, in these areas, all are the same. However, there are distinct differences among the four. Look at the italicized information to remember the differences among the four types.*

**Scholarship of Discovery.** Examples are peer-reviewed publications of research, theory, or philosophical essays, and grant awards in support of research or scholarship. Discovery includes *primary empirical research, historical research, theory development, and testing.* It includes state, regional, national, and international recognition.

**Scholarship of Teaching.** Examples are peer-reviewed publications of research related to *teaching methodology or learning outcomes* and grant awards in support of teaching and learning. It includes state, regional national international recognition.

**Scholarship of Practice (Application).** Examples are peer-reviewed publications of research, case studies, *technical applications or other practice issues* and grant awards in support of practice. It includes state, regional national international recognition.

**Scholarship of Integration.** Examples are peer-reviewed publications of research, policy analysis, case studies, integrative reviews of literature, interdisciplinary grant awards, *copyrights, licenses, patents, or products for sale.*

### Developing Mnemonic Devices

Develop mnemonics if a memory aid is needed; however, using mnemonics may be less useful in some situations where it may be easier to just remember the facts. For example, when the nurse educator is developing a test, the BOBCAT mnemonic can provide guidance to develop the test appropriately. This mnemonic stands for:

- **B**lueprint
- **O**bjectives of the course
- **B**loom's Taxonomy
- **C**lient Needs Categories (NCLEX-RN)
- **A**nalysis Data
- **T**est Results and Changes for the Future

In summary: A **B**lueprint is developed from the **O**bjectives of the course. **B**loom's Taxonomy is used to develop questions in higher cognitive levels such as application and analysis. **C**lient Needs Categories of NCLEX-RN® are necessary to guide faculty to construct questions in the eight categories, such as Management of Care, Safety and Infection Control, Health Promotion and Maintenance, and Reduction of Risk Potential to name a few (see chapter 4, Table 4.4). **A**nalysis of data is performed and **T**est results are determined. After the results of the test are reviewed, revisions to items should be completed so they can be used in the future.

## Relate New Information to Be Learned to Information Already Mastered

Learning new information is easier if it can be related to information or facts that are already understood. An example of this learning strategy is illustrated here: Many times test validity and test reliability become confused. If you understand what test validity means, *you only need to add to your memory the information about reliability.*

- *Validity* means the test is measuring the information it is supposed to measure. It is "valid." The test blueprint is used to developed questions related to the objectives of the course; this ensures validity.
- *Reliability* refers to the consistency of the test scores. The test's reliability can be improved by making changes to the items so that they are more discriminating.

### Correlate Testing With Practice

Examine your own activities as an educator and relate them to the content in the questions. This will be helpful in developing a complete understanding of the information. You will find that your experience will be very helpful in answering questions. Many examples of how to correlate your own experience with the content to be learned are presented in Exhibit 1.2.

| Exhibit 1.2 | Relating Question Content to Educator Experience |

| Question Content | Educator Experience |
| --- | --- |
| Create opportunities for the learners to develop their own critical thinking skills. | Students can develop critical thinking skills by participating in the following assignments: writing a teaching plan, developing a concept map, completing an exercise in delegation or prioritization in the clinical area, or utilizing a case study in the simulation laboratory. |
| Use information technologies to support the teaching-learning process. | Specific materials may be taught more effectively by using technology. It may be advantageous for specific learners to use video streaming, Blackboard ™ discussions, synchronous discussions, or Web-enhanced classes. |
| Respond effectively to unexpected events that affect the clinical and/or classroom instruction. | Collect all the information, including anecdotal records if it occurred at the clinical site. Clarify professional behavior as outlined in the Code of Ethics for Nurses with Interpretive Statement and Nursing: Scope and Standards of Practice.<br>Utilize conflict resolution, if indicated. Refer the student to the Student Conduct Committee, if indicated. |
| Identify learning styles and unique learning needs of students from culturally diverse backgrounds. | Many students speak English as a second language (ESL). The development of communication and active learning in the classroom may assist with understanding of information such as:<br>1. Discussing cultural beliefs related to a specific disease, since this can impact client care in the clinical setting.<br>2. Answering questions during class in pairs or small groups.<br>3. Reviewing questions using clickers to improve class participation.<br>4. Playing Jeopardy in the classroom. |
| Provide input for the development of nursing program standards and policies regarding:<br>1. Admission<br>2. Progression<br>3. Graduation | If you have not had the opportunity to work with the admissions, academic progression, or graduation committees in your college of nursing, then request permission to review the minutes or attend meetings. Involvement in these committees promotes a clear understanding of the process.<br>Admission criteria are usually posted on the school's Web site and include SAT scores, entrance examination scores, GPA, and Test of English as a Foreign Language (TOEFL) requirements for students born in non-English-speaking countries. |

*(Continued)*

| Exhibit 1.2 | Relating Question Content to Educator Experience (Continued) |
| --- | --- |

| Question Content | Educator Experience |
| --- | --- |
| | The progression committee determines if a student should be permitted to continue in the program after failure of a course or courses. The committee may overturn a decision if the student had extenuating circumstances, such as a serious illness or death in the family. The students may also go through the academic appeals process to overturn a grade they believe to be inaccurate. The committee also takes into account the student's grades in prerequisite and co-requisite courses when making a decision. Graduation occurs when the student completes the minimum number of credits specified for the degree and his or her GPA is within the program standards. A student must also complete the clinical requirements for courses with a satisfactory rating in the clinical component. |
| Participate in curriculum development or revision. | Read and compare the mission statements and philosophy statements of the university and the college of nursing. Review the level objectives and the behavioral objectives in the nursing program curriculum. Level objectives are reflective of the progressive competence of the students within the goals and philosophy of the program. Behavioral objectives drive the design for the courses, with a focus on learning outcomes. The curriculum is updated as needed to incorporate changes in the student body and the community, the use of technology, and current health care trends. The goal is to improve program outcomes. |
| Use feedback gained from self, peer, and learner evaluations to improve role effectiveness. | Self-evaluation can assist faculty members in determining their own needs, such as: preparation for class, organization of teaching strategy, and test development. Student opinions are important because students spend many hours in class. Students may have a need for the enhancement of information or clinical opportunities that are not recognized by the educator. Student evaluations can be used to improve the course. |

*(Continued)*

| Exhibit 1.2 | Relating Question Content to Educator Experience (Continued) |

| Question Content | Educator Experience |
| --- | --- |
| | Peer evaluations can be helpful, however they can also cause conflict between faculty members. The faculty should have specific guidelines designated for the evaluation and the date of the didactic evaluation should be decided by both faculty members. |
| Use legal and ethical principles to influence, design, and implement policies and procedures related to learners, faculty, and the educational environment. | Legal issues can include: 1. Co-signing documentation in the clinical area 2. Providing care that results in an injury to the client or the student 3. Completion of an incident report 4. Cheating during an examination 5. Plagiarism on a class assignment 6. Dismissal of a student from the program The college should have policies addressing these issues. In addition, students are protected by the U.S. Constitution's Bill of Rights: The First Amendment protects freedom of religion, press, speech, and the right to assemble. The Fourth Amendment provides protection against unreasonable search and seizure. |
| Use evidence-based resources to improve and support teaching. | Evidenced-based resources can be used in the classroom or clinical setting by: 1. Scheduling an assignment in which one group of students takes a turn discussing a research article related to the content presented in the classroom that week. 2. Providing evidence-based articles to students in the clinical module who have down time. The student(s) will take time to review the article and present the information during post conference. |
| Participate in departmental and institutional committees. | Examples of committees within the nursing department include: faculty affairs, student affairs, scholarship and innovation, faculty resources, and technology. Some examples of committees within an institution include: faculty and governance, faculty finance, green team |

# References

American Academy of Colleges of Nursing. (2009). Retrieved January 11, 2009, from http://www.aacn.nche.edu/Media/FactSheets/NursingShortage.htm

Cranton, P. (2002). Teaching for transformation. *New Direction for Adult and Continuing Education, 93,* 63–71.

Meizrow, J. (1991). *Transformative dimensions of adult learning.* San Francisco: Jossey-Bass.

National League for Nursing (NLN). (2009a). *Certified Nurse Educator (CNE) Detailed Test Blueprint.* Retrieved March 25, 2009, from http://www.nln.org/facultycertification/index.htm

National League for Nursing (NLN). (2009b). *Certified Nurse Educator (CNE) 2009 Candidate Handbook.* Retrieved March 28, 2009, from http://www.nln.org/facultycertification/handbook/cne.pdf

Neese, R. (2003). A transformational journey from clinical to educator. *The Journal of Continuing Education in Nursing, 34*(6), 258–262.

U.S. Bureau of Labor Statistics. (2007). *Registered nurses.* Retrieved March 29, 2009, from http://www.bls.gov/oco/ocos083.htm

Yordy, K. D. (2006). *The nursing faculty shortage: A crisis for healthcare.* Princeton, NJ: Robert Wood Johnson Foundation.

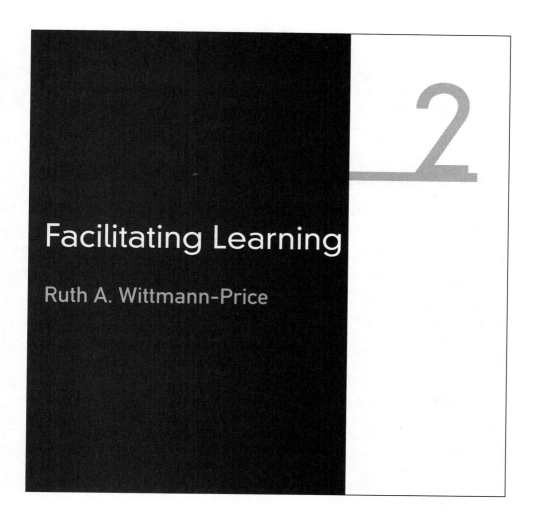

# Facilitating Learning

Ruth A. Wittmann-Price

*Strive for excellence, not perfection.*

—H. Jackson Brown, Jr.

**NLN Core Competency I: Facilitate Learning**

Nurse educators are responsible for creating an environment in the classroom, laboratory and clinical settings that facilitates student learning and the achievement of desired cognitive, affective and psychomotor outcomes (National League for Nursing [NLN], 2005, p. 15).

**Learning Outcomes**

- Discuss the theoretical and philosophical underpinnings of nursing education.
- Interpret methods that assess learners' styles and needs.
- Comprehend the components of a teaching/learning plan.

■ Evaluate the teaching style that you use most.

■ Synthesize methodologies into your present teaching/learning environment that will enhance critical thinking and metacognition.

## Introduction

Nursing education today is more exciting and challenging than ever before. Gone are the days of a homogenous classroom of students who respond unquestioningly to lock-step teaching and learning methods. Now nurse educators facilitate learning for students of all ages, from many different lifestyles, ethnic and cultural backgrounds, with different generational characteristics, and most importantly, different learning styles. The overarching goal is that every student deserves nurse educators who best can facilitate his or her journey toward becoming a successful, professional nurse. Education expertise is needed to assist students to pass the NCLEX-RN exam. Perhaps most importantly, faculty must facilitate the development of critical thinking skills and inspire the love of lifelong learning in order to prepare nursing professionals who can provide the best care for patients and enjoy a rewarding and fulfilling career.

## Educational Philosophies

Educational philosophies are never stagnant, they change as the larger social system matures, but they nonetheless provide the foundations on which educational pedagogies are built. It is the academic institution's educational philosophy from which the *mission statement,* the curriculum, learning outcomes, and teaching theories are derived (Csokasy, 2005). Nursing's educational philosophies date back to Florence Nightingale, who can be credited with the first nursing education philosophy. Below are summations of the major educational philosophies and some of their salient features. *What belief(s) speak to you as a nursing educator?*

### Traditional Philosophies

■ *Idealism*

  ■ People would like to live in a perfect world.

■ *Realism*

  ■ The world is orderly, and science can be viewed objectively and analyzed.

■ *Essentialism* (Plato, Aristotle)

  ■ A traditional education approach that develops students' minds through knowledge passed to the student from the teacher.
  ■ A core curriculum is valued, as are democracy and cultural heritage.
  ■ The physical world is the true reality; students should appreciate the masterworks of art and literature.

- Students need critical thinking skills to help society.
- Teacher-directed learning.

- *Perennialism* (Thomas Aquinas)

  - Traditional education style that is teacher-centered.
  - Liberal education is valued.
  - Studies should include great thinkers of the past but also prepare students for adult life.
  - Reading, writing, and arithmetic are important.

- *Behaviorism* (Pavlov, Watson, Skinner)

  - Stimuli-response is the basis for learning.
  - The environment develops the person.
  - Requires behavior modification and classroom management.
  - Positive reinforcement is used to encourage acceptable behavior.
  - Generated the idea of "Programmed Learning."
  - Tyler (1949) refers to this philosophy as the one that introduced behavioral objectives (see the section in Chapter 2 on learning objectives vs. learning outcomes in education).
  - Faculty decides about the educational experience.
  - Nursing education is still steeped in behaviorism (lock-step curriculum) today.

## Modern Philosophies and Postmodern Philosophies

- *Pragmatism*

  - Ideas can be tested scientifically.
  - The human experience is important.
  - Influenced by social reform and the growth of citizenship in early 19th century.

- *Reconstructionism*

  - School is important for social change.
  - School alone can prepare a student for life.

- *Progressivism* (John Dewey)

  - School mimics society.
  - Real-life curriculum and problem-solving exercises are the most important aspects of education.
  - Attend to and optimize the inquisitive, active learning style of children.
  - Experiential learning takes place in the classroom.
  - Students have choices about what to learn.
  - Students are engaged in group and peer learning.
  - Education experiences are student-centered.

- *Existentialism* (Kierkegaard, Buber, May, Rogers, Neill)
    - Seeks individual meaning in life.
    - Schools hold social ideals.
    - Perception of the individual is reality.
    - No one can know us as we know ourselves.
    - Education of the whole person is the goal.
    - Subject matter takes second place to the development of a positive self concept, self knowledge, and self responsibility.
    - Students have great latitude in choosing subject matter.

- *Phenomenological* (Heidegger)
    - Hermeneutical analysis.
    - Knowledge development comes through dialogue and reflection.
    - Based on an empowering and liberating framework where knowledge is discovered.

- *Humanism* (Rogers, Maslow)
    - Human beings are autonomous and the dignity of human beings is the most important thing in the world.
    - Self-actualization and education lead to individual happiness.
    - A nursing approach can be found in Bevis and Watson's "The caring curriculum" (1989).

- *Feminism*
    - Personal knowledge is true knowledge.
    - Power in the classroom must be analyzed.
    - No human being should be marginalized.
    - Places a great emphasis on empowerment and the students' voices (Weyenberg, 1998).
    - Empirical knowledge is only one type of knowledge (Berragan, 1998).

- *Narrative Pedagogy* (Diekelmann & Scheckel, 2004)
    - Focus is on the meaning and significance of teaching through phenomenology pedagogies such as storytelling.
    - Builds experiences that stray from a formal, competency-based, outcome education format. This approach supports the development of deeper thinking and meaning in lived experiences.

- *Emancipatory Education* (Freire, 1970)
    - Education is a microsystem of society.
    - Teachers are cultural workers who profess freedom though an equalized classroom.
    - Teachers and students are both learners through true dialogue. (Philosophies adapted from: Csokasy, 2005; Ellsworth, 1998; Wittmann-Price, 2007.)

- *Critical Pedagogy* (Vickers, 2008)
    - Includes concepts from feminism, phenomenology, and critical social theory.

- Phenomenology—Gain greater understanding in the human experience.
- Critical social theory—Liberation from oppressive structures is essential to well being.
- Feminism—Gender biases exist.

## Learning Theories

How students learn and how they store, connect, discover, and retrieve skills and information has been well studied and formalized into many theoretical frameworks. These frameworks try to explain the connection between knowledge and the human brain, a truly interesting subject that affects us and our students every day.

Educational philosophy guides learning theories, and there is some overlap in terms and ideas from one theory to the next. Philosophies are driven by *metaphysics,* or the study of what is real, *epistemology,* what is knowledge and truth, and *axiology,* what is good (Csokasy, 2005). Theories have more defined concepts and are more applicable to the teaching situation. All learning theories fall into three categories: behaviorism, cognitivism, and constructivism.

### Behaviorism

- Learning is observable through behavior.
- Learning is reinforced by response.
- Behavior modification leads to control.
- Token economies may be used for classroom management.
- Instructional objectives guide learning (Tyler, 1949).
- Behaviorism does not explain the intrinsic motivations of the learner.
- Learning is shaped by others.
- Teacher-centered.
- Behaviorists: Watson, Skinner, Pavlov, Bandura

  - *Bandura*—Social Learning Theory (Kessler et al., 1995).

    - Perception of confidence in oneself in the situation (self-efficacy).
    - Self-efficacy is based on four principles:

      - Enactive mastery experiences, or the learner's own history of successes.
      - Vicarious experiences, or the observed behaviors of a role model being successful at a task.
      - Verbal persuasion, or telling someone they will be successful.
      - Physiological states, or the person's "gut feeling" that they can succeed.

    - Positive expectations are the incentives. Bandura's term, reciprocal determinism, meaning that the world and the person's behavior cause each other.

### Cognitivism, or Information Processing Theories

- Learning is a function of the brain (sometimes called brain-based learning).
- Describes how information is received, stored, and processed in the mind.
- Humans process information and store it in memory.
- Memory is achieved by sensory input, which goes to short-term memory (working memory), which is then stored, if significant, in long-term memory, in which information may be forgotten but is never lost completely.
- Encoding and relating incoming information to old information makes it more memorable.
- Student-centered.
- Gagne's (1970) nine events of instruction are shown in Table 2.1.

### Constructivism

- Learning is built by the learner
- Learning is actively constructed through interaction with the environment, and it is marked by reflection and actions.

| Table 2.1 | Gagne's Nine Events of Instruction |
|---|---|
| **Instructional Event** | **Internal Process That Goes on in the Brain** |
| 1. Gain attention of the student | Stimuli activates receptors |
| 2. Inform learners of objectives | Sets expectations for the learner |
| 3. Stimulate recall of prior learning | Activate short-term memory and the retrieval of information by asking questions |
| 4. Present the content | Present content with features that can be remembered |
| 5. Provide "learning guidance" | Assist the learner to organize the information for long-term memory |
| 6. Elicit performance (practice) | Ask learners to perform to enhance encoding and verification |
| 7. Provide appropriate feedback | Encourage performance |
| 8. Assess performance | Evaluate |
| 9. Enhance retention and transfer | Review periodically to decrease memory loss of information |

Adapted from *Psychology of Learning for Instruction* (2nd ed.), by M. P. Driscoll, 2000. Needham Heights, MA: Allyn & Bacon and *Gagne's Nine Events of Instruction: An Introduction*, by K. Kruse, n.d. Retrieved August 2, 2008, from http://www.e-learningguru.com/articles/art3_3.htm.

- The learner tries to make sense out of his or her experiences.
- The goal is for problem solving, reasoning, critical thinking, and the active and reflective use of knowledge that does not have to resemble the environment.
- What the learner perceives is most important.
- Student-focused.
- Piaget, Bruner, Vygotsky
- Constructivists' conditions of learning (Driscoll, 2000) include:

  - Learning should be embedded in a realistic environment
  - Social negotiation is a part of learning.
  - Support multiple perspectives on subjects.
  - Taking ownership of learning is important
  - Be self-aware and reflective in the knowledge acquisition process. (Learning Theories adapted from Driscoll, 2000; Chinn, 2007).

## Deep Learning

Deep learning is a term first described by Marton and Saljo (1976) to refer to a learning approach and type of knowledge acquisition (Ross & Tuovinen, 2001). The approach a student takes to information presented in the classroom can be classified into three types of learning styles: deep, surface, and strategic.

- A deep learning approach is accomplished when a student addresses material with the intent to understand both the concepts and meaning of the information.

  - These students relate new ideas to existing experiences.
  - Formulate links in long-term memory.
  - The motivation for a deep learning approach is primarily intrinsic, created from the student's interest and desire to understand the relevance of the information to applied practice (McMahon, 2006).

- A surface learning, or atomistic, approach facilitates learning by the:

  - Memorization of facts and details. Surface learning is similar to rote learning in that the student assimilates information presented at face value (Diseth, 2002).
  - Motivation for surface learning is primarily extrinsic, driven either by the student's fear of failing or by the student's desire to complete the course successfully (McMahon, 2006).

- A third learning approach is called strategic learning. Using this learning approach, the student does what is needed to complete a course. Strategic learning is a mixture of both deep and surface learning techniques (Cowan et al., 2004).
- All three approaches to learning can be measured by the Approaches to Student Inventory (ASSIST) (Entwistle, 1999; Ramsden & Entwistle, 1981).

## Motivational Theories

Not only do educators need to know how students learn, they also need to know why they learn. What is the motivating factor? Motivation is goal-directed behavior and, according to Schunk and Zimmerman (1994), it is reciprocal with self-regulatory skills. A learner must not only be motivated, he or she must also have self-regulatory skills to sustain and achieve the goals of education (Driscoll, 2000). Many variables effect motivation; it can be influenced by the need for achievement or curiosity, or it can be a function of the situation at hand or a person's ability. Another factor is the student's locus of control whether the motivation is extrinsic or intrinsic. Positive expectations with parents and educators serve as incentives to motivation. There are also variables that produce a lack of motivation, such as lack of expectations and anxiety.

### Self-Efficacy

Self-efficacy, or a person's belief about the capabilities of their behavior, is also interwoven with a student's motivation (Bandura, 1997). According to Bandura, self-efficacy is developed in the following four ways:

- Enactive, mastery experiences, or if the student has been successful at something before.
- Vicarious experiences, or the student observing a role model being successful at a learning skill.
- Verbal persuasion, or someone encouraging the learner to succeed.
- Physiological states, or the student's intrinsic judging of his or her own ability.

Motivation is generally discussed in *extrinsic* and *intrinsic* forms. Intrinsic motivation has to do with the feeling of accomplishment, of learning for the sake of learning, while extrinsic motivation is related to rewards outside the individual.

Keller (1987) talks about the factors educators can implement to motivate students in the *ARCS model:*

A = Attention (keeping the student's attention through stimulus changes in the classroom or clinical setting)
R = Relevance (make the information relevant to the student's goals)
C = Confidence (make expectations clear so the students will engage in learning)
S = Satisfaction (have appropriate consequences for the students' new skills)

Brophy (1986) listed the following methods by which motivation is formed:

- Modeling
- Communication of expectations
- Direct instruction
- Socialization by parents and teachers

Levett-Jones and Lathlean (2008) studied the concept of *belongingness* in nursing students related to clinical learning and determined that it is conceptually related to the motivation to learn. The themes identified in students about learning are listed in Exhibit 2.1.

Lottes (2008) uses a formula that she calls *fire up* to enhance students' classroom motivation. This motivational strategy is shown in Exhibit 2.2.

DeYoung (2003) lists 10 principles to motivate learners (p. 62); they are applicable not only to patients but also to students:

- Use several senses
- Actively involve the learner
- Assess readiness
- Determine if the learner thinks the information is relevant
- Repeat information
- Generalize information
- Make learning pleasant
- Begin with what is known
- Present information at an appropriate rate
- Provide a learning-friendly environment

*What was your motivation for going back to school to become a nurse educator or for studying for the CNE?*

| Exhibit 2.1 | Themes Specific to Belongingness and Learning |
|---|---|

Theme A = Motivation to learn—being accepted and valued as a student
Theme B = Self-directed learning (SDL) assists in building confidence
Theme C = Anxiety—a barrier to learning
Theme D = Confidence to ask questions

| Exhibit 2.2 | Lottes' FIRE-UP Motivational Strategy |
|---|---|

| | |
|---|---|
| F | Be Funny—use light entertainment to increase attention. |
| I | Be Interesting—Use graphics to help students focus. |
| R | Be Real—Remember that you were a nursing student once. |
| E | Engage them—use active learning techniques. |
| U | Be Unique—Use an individual style in the classroom. |
| P | Be Passionate—Of course, love what you do. |

## Change Theories

Learning takes motivation, and that motivation actually assists a person seeking to change either cognitively or behaviorally. Change and motivation are interwoven concepts; each is dependent on the other. Change (learning new information, skills, or affects) does not happen unless a student is motivated; therefore, an unmotivated student most likely will not change. A brief description of popular change theories are outlined in Table 2.2. (For further information about change theories, please see Chapter 5.)

## Pedagogy

Pedagogy is generally defined as the art and science of teaching. It refers to the manner in which educators instruct. Instruction can be accomplished through the use of many styles that often are closely aligned with the educational philosophy on which they are based. Table 2.3 displays some common pedagogies and their characteristics.

## Andragogy

Two of the most compared teaching praxis in nursing are pedagogy and andragogy. Andragogy is generally defined as teaching strategies useful when teaching

| Table 2.2 | Theoretical Constructs About Change |
|---|---|
| **Theory** | **Major Paradigm** |
| Transtheoretical Model (TM) | Five stages and 10 processes of change. Stages include pre-contemplation, contemplation, preparation; action and maintenance to get ready for change. Ten processes are behavior activities that support the stage (Humphreys, Thompson, & Miner, 1998). |
| Theory of Reasoned Action (TRA) | Reasoned action theorizes that actual behavior is determined by intention that includes both attitudes and subjective norms (Manstead, Proffitt, & Smart, 1983). |
| Theory of Planned Behavior (TPB) | Behavior is determined by intention and ability (Swanson & Power, 2005). |
| Bandura's Social Learning Theory (self-efficacy) | Perception of confidence in oneself (Bandura, 1997). |
| Social Cognitive Theory | This theory is based on reciprocity between the individual, environment, and personal factors. If one is changed, they all are changed (DeYoung, 2003). |
| Behavior Modification Theory | This theory works on the reward and punishment system to promote change (DeYoung, 2003). |

| Table 2.3 | Common Pedagogies |
|-----------|-------------------|

| Type of Pedagogy | Characteristics of Pedagogy |
|------------------|------------------------------|
| Andragogy | Commonly associated with Malcolm Knowles' (1984) theory although its roots date back to the 1980s (Milligan, 1995). Key elements are self-directed adult learning that builds on life experiences. It promotes autonomy and critical thinking |
| Interpretive pedagogies Phenomenological (pedagogy that is interpretative and transformative through narrative, understanding, and dialogue), critical (understanding through dialogue, critique, comparison, and contrast), feminist (discovering how gender shapes thinking and how to emancipate), and postmodern (discovers the power of politics and creating a voice) (Diekelmann, 1995). | Call for a reawakening in thinking about how nursing is taught. Diekelmann (1988) describes it as "teaching as uncovering learning." |
| Feminist pedagogy | Hezekiah (1993) proposed five major concepts in feminist pedagogy: Mutual respect, trust and community, shared leadership, cooperative environment, integration of cognitive and affective learning, and action oriented learning or praxis |
| Pedagogy | The basis of pedagogy, according to Van Manen (1991), is to mimic a parenting relationship that is based in practical application. It is situational and normative and assists the student to develop and grow. |

adult learners. Table 2.4 shows more distinct differences between andragogy and pedagogy.

## Assessing the Learner and the Teacher

### Assessing the Learner

Many clinical nursing courses are content laden. Furthermore, the sizes of classes have increased exponentially in the past decade. Because of these two

| Table 2.4 | Andragogy and Pedagogy | |
|---|---|---|
| | **Andragogy** | **Pedagogy** |
| *Demands of learning* | Students have life demands besides school. | Student can devote more time to the demands of learning because responsibilities are minimal. |
| *Role of instructor* | Students are autonomous and self-directed. Teachers facilitate the students' learning, but don't supply all the facts. | Teacher-centered because the teacher directs the learning. Often uses surface learning. |
| *Life experiences* | Students have a tremendous amount of life experience. They need to connect the learning to their knowledge base. They must recognize the value of the learning. | Students do not have the knowledge base to make the connections of new knowledge to life experiences without facilitation. |
| *Purpose for learning* | Students have a goal in sight for their learning. | Students cannot always see the long term necessity of information. |
| *Permanence of learning* | Learning is self-initiated and tends to last a long time. | Learning is compulsory and tends to disappear shortly after instruction. |

Adapted from "Andragogy: Teaching Adults," by J. Green, 1998, in B. Hoffman (Ed.), *Encyclopedia of Educational Technology.*

characteristics, it is challenging for nursing faculty to provide learning experiences that meet the needs of the variety of learning styles for all students in a class, especially considering that those learning styles may vary depending on the type of information presented in the class. Therefore, it is helpful to assess learning styles for the purpose of planning appropriate content presentations. Learning styles can be assessed according to Curry Onion's Model of Learning and Cognitive Style (Polhemus et al., 2005) which maintains that there are four components that make up a learning style. These include:

- The personality dimensions of the student
- The way the student processes information
- The way in which a student perceives him or herself in the classroom
- Multidimensional and instructional preference models, which include:
  - Environmental factors
  - Teaching strategies that the student prefers

These components can be used to categorize learning styles. There are a variety of ways that have been developed to do this. One, by Honey and Mumford (2006), categorizes learners into four types of learning styles:

- Reflector
- Theorist
- Pragmatist
- Activist

Another, Filipczak (1995), identifies learning styles in relation to sensory intake, a categorization that is better known in the educational world. The three categories include:

- Auditory
- Kinesthetic and tactile
- Visual

A third approach to categorizing learning styles is through generational differences (Johnson & Romanello, 2005). A great deal of current literature focuses on generational differences that result from style of child-rearing practices, the technological infusion of society, and the political presences during the students' developing years. Table 2.5 presents the generational differences in student character and teaching strategies that can be adapted to facilitate learning for the various generational groups.

Lastly, learning styles of students can be classified according to the type of educational program in which students are enrolled. Students who are traditional high school graduates entering an Associate or Baccalaureate program will likely differ in learning style from students who are second career nursing students on an accelerated path to becoming an RN. There has been a deluge of literature on the learning differences of the second degree learner compared to the traditional college-age student, even though they may be from the same generation category. Table 2.6 outlines some differences between the perspectives of adult learners and traditional college-aged learners. Note that further information on learning styles of students can be found in Chapter 3.

## Developing Teaching Strategies to Meet the Learning Needs of Students

### Accelerated Students

Developed due to the nursing shortage, second-degree or accelerated nursing programs range from 11 to 15 months. Many different indicators have been used to admit, retain, and graduate the second degree learner. Bentley (2006) found that the students' science grade point average (GPA) was predictive of success.

## Evidence-Based Education

A literature review by Chauvin (2008) states that nurse educators must take into account two differences with second degree accelerated students. The first is that they are different than the traditional students; the faculty cannot ignore this. The second difference is that their prior learning is not always a guarantee of success. Some accelerated students have developed learning habits that are inflexible.

**Table 2.5 — Generational Differences That Characterize Learners Today**

| Generational Label | What Students Expect | What Facilitates Learning |
|---|---|---|
| Born between 1946 and 1964 *"Baby Boomer" generation* | Most faculty, average age is 45.2–51 (Mangold, 2007; Arhin & Cormiere, 2007; Walker et al., 2008) | ■ Large peer group (80 million strong) increases competition (Mangold, 2007). <br>■ Taught mainly by lecture; thinks technology is nice to have, but not essential. |
| Born between 1965 and 1979 *"Generation X"* | ■ Challenge authority. <br>■ Independent problem solvers and multitaskers. | ■ Self-learning modules <br>■ Demonstration and return demo <br>■ Pragmatic and focus on the outcomes of learning not the process <br>■ Want real world skills |
| Born after 1975 or between 1981 and 1999 (Mangold, 2007) <br>May be labeled: <br>*"Generation Y'ers"* <br>*"Millennials"* <br>*"Nexters"* <br>*"MTV Generation"* <br><br>*This generation is:* <br>■ More culturally diverse <br>■ One third raised in single parent homes <br>■ 81 million strong (Walker et al., 2008) | ■ Constant stimulation <br>■ Multimedia and instant information critical consumers; expect entertainment <br>■ Active learners <br>■ Hands on learning <br>■ Fast-paced experience <br>■ Instant gratification <br>■ Positive reinforcement <br>■ Resourceful <br>■ Challenge of problem-solving <br>■ Group activities <br><br>*Some shared characteristics:* <br>■ Poor reading and math skills <br>■ Poor work habits <br>■ Multitaskers <br>■ No time for school <br>■ Visual learners due to computers | ■ Critical reading <br>■ Intertextuality: reading from multiple sources to critically appraise the overlap for meaning <br>■ Self-preferentiality: better critiquing if it is a topic they are passionate about or can relate to in their own lives <br>■ Reading from different positions: considering different viewpoints or cultural interpretations <br>■ Journaling to foster reflection and critical thinking <br>■ Encourage using technology to write through peer evaluation <br>■ Concept mapping (Arhin & Cormiere, 2007) Simulation in teams (Mangold, 2007; Pardue & Morgan, 2008) |

| Table 2.6 | Comparing Characteristics of Second-Degree Learners to Traditional College Learners |
|---|---|

| Traditional College-age Learners | Second-career Learners |
|---|---|
| Technologically savvy | View education more critically (Bradshaw & Nugent, 1997) |
| Task driven | Sophisticated consumers |
| Teachers are authoritarian figures | Goal-oriented (Bradshaw & Nugent, 1997) |
| More educational resources from being on campus | Have sacrificed financially and socially (Wittmann-Price, 2007) |

## BSN Students

Another educational consideration is the BSN student, or RN to BSN, who has a diploma or Associates degree in nursing. There is discussion about requiring nurses to have a BSN degree within ten years of their generic degree (RN plus 10). There is also a call for multiple program options, rather than regimented coursework and a focus on evidence-based nursing practice. Community and leadership also may need to be redesigned to meet the needs of this ever-increasing student population, one that brings wonderful experience to the educational arena (Speakman, DeRaineri, & Schaal, 2008).

## The Male Nursing Student

Increasing numbers of men are entering nursing. Five to six percent of U.S. men work in nursing (Wolfe, 2007), and 5.7% of nurses are men (Nelson, 2006). This is a 226% increase since 1980 (Grady, Stewardson, & Hall, 2008). As nursing students, men may experience stereotyping or experience gender bias by nurse educators. It is important for faculty to be aware that male nursing students have the right to a non-discriminating educational experience. Grady (2008) studied men in nursing and identified aspects of caring as a concept identified in male caregivers. Gender differences create challenges that are only now being addressed by faculty and, increasingly, being overcome. One particular challenge for men in this female-dominated career is that their sexual orientation may be questioned. Such challenges are considered educational or work-place discrimination. It is important for faculty to work toward eliminating discriminatory behavior in the educational environment; this is especially important as the profession increases in diversity and moves forward. As Wolfe (2007) explains,

> Most of the misconceptions come from families, for instance, the first time they see me, they assume I'm a doctor, when I correct them, they ask me why I didn't become one. I tell them being a nurse allows me to focus on fewer patients so I can spend more time at the bedside and get to know them better, I'm exactly where I want to be. (p. 12)

Nelson (2006) describes public campaigns to change the stereotypical image of men in nursing and attempts to foster recruitment efforts.

# Evidence-Based Education

Loughrey (2008) studied male nurses' sex role perceptions ($N = 104$) in Ireland. He used the short-form Berm Sex Role Inventory, and found 78 respondents identified nursing as a more feminine than masculine role. This study defined gender as socio-cultural construct with certain expectations, roles, and behaviors. Further studies are needed on gender roles and cultural perceptions.

## Using Learning Style Assessments to Facilitate Learning Outcomes

### Assessing Learning Styles

Knowing a learner's learning style will assist the teacher to maximize the student's learning experience. Some learning needs and parameters to assess include (Brancato, 2007):

- Learning needs, or the internal motivation for learning.
- Readiness to learn
  - Interest
  - Receptivity (Bastable, 2007)
    - Barriers to readiness (Brancato, 2007)
      - Emotions
      - Anxiety
      - Experiential
      - Cultural
      - Language
- Developmental stage
- Motivation—the will and desire (Davis, 1993)
- Emotional intelligence (EI)—intrapersonal and interpersonal skills in:
  - Self-awareness
  - Self-regulation
  - Social awareness
  - Self-motivation
  - Social skills (Freshman & Rubino, 2002)
- Literacy assessment
  - Readability
  - Comprehension (Brancato, 2007) (For further information about student learning styles, please see Chapter 3).

## Tools for Assessing Students' Learning Styles

There are many learning style assessment tools that can be employed for the purpose of improving faculty understanding of the mix of learning styles within a student group. This information can then be used to determine the best teaching modalities to use with the group. Learning style assessment also can be utilized for remediation, tutoring, or counseling students (Brancato, 2007).

Some of the more commonly used assessment tools include:

- The Kolb Learning Style Inventory (Kolb, 1976) places the student into one of four learning styles:

  - Accommodative—prefers concrete experience and active experimentation
  - Assimilative—prefers abstract conceptualization and reflective observation
  - Divergent—prefers concrete experience and reflective observation
  - Convergent—prefers abstract conceptualization and active experimentation

- Dunn, Dunn, and Price Productivity Environmental Preference Survey (PEPS) (1996) is a self-diagnostic instrument and assesses four categories:

  - Environmental—preference for light, noise, temperature, etc.
  - Sociological—preference for studying alone or in groups
  - Physical—visual, auditory, or kinesthetic
  - Emotional—responsibility, persistence, and motivation

- The VARK inventory is an online assessment for auditory, visual, or kinesthetic preferences in learning (Fleming, 2009). The VARK can be found at http://www.vark-learn.com/english/index.asp and further information is in Chapter 3.

## Critical Thinking Questions

Which teaching strategies are you most comfortable with? Which are more compatible with a humanistic orientation, a psychoanalytical approach, or a cognitive orientation?

## Assessing Faculty Teaching Styles

Teaching style is another variable that contributes to the effectiveness of teaching in the class and the clinical area. There are many ways to classify teaching style. Teaching styles have also been categorized differently by various educational researchers and experts.

## Grasha's Classification

Grasha's (1996) classification defines teaching styles as expert, formal authority, demonstrator, facilitator, and delegator. The characteristics of each teaching style are unique and are listed in Table 2.7.

## Quirk's Classification

Quirk (1994) categorizes teaching styles into four distinct types:

- Assertive—An assertive style is usually content-specific and drives home a piece of information.
- Suggestive—The teacher uses experiences to describe a concept and then requests the students research more information on the subject.
- Collaborative—The teacher uses skills to promote problem solving and a higher level of thinking in the students.
- Facilitative—Teachers using this style often challenge the students to reflect and use affective learning. They challenge them to ask ethical questions and to demonstrate skill with interpersonal relationships and professional behavior.

Teachers rarely ascribe to just one teaching style. Most teachers use a variety of styles, even within a single teaching-learning session. This mixed approach can appeal to the variety of student learning styles and improve learning outcomes. A teacher's tendency toward one style or several of the above styles can be evaluated using learning assessment tools found on the Web. Reflecting on the type of style that you use most encourages self-understanding and may serve to improve your own teaching effectiveness.

| Table 2.7 | Teaching Styles Characterized by Grasha |
|---|---|
| **Style** | **Characteristics** |
| Expert | Uses their vast knowledge base to inform students and challenges them to be well prepared. This can be intimidating to the student. |
| Formal Authority | This style puts the teacher in control of the students' knowledge acquisition. The teacher is not concerned with student-teacher relationships, but rather focuses on the content to be delivered. |
| Demonstrator or Personal Model | The teacher coaches, demonstrates, and encourages a more active student learning style. |
| Facilitator | Student-centered, active learning strategies are encouraged. The accountability for learning is placed on the learner. |
| Delegator | The teacher role is that of a consultant and the students are encouraged to direct the entire learning project. |

## Teaching Behaviors

Individual teaching styles involve teaching behaviors and are noteworthy because behaviors have a direct effect on the teaching-learning environment. House, Chassie, and Spohn (1999) provide examples of the following behaviors and their effect on students:

- Making *eye contact* can encourage student participation in class.
- Positive facial expressions that elicit a positive student response, such as head nodding, can assist students in feeling comfortable dialoguing in class, whereas negative gestures, such as frowning, can discourage student class participation.
- Vocal tone is very important and can easily portray underlying feelings and encourage or discourage student participation.

## Personal Attributes That Facilitate Learning

A teaching style is a mixture of the teacher's personality and learned educational skills in the classroom and clinical area. Many authors speak about the attributes that facilitate a positive learning environment. There is little doubt that the teacher establishes much of that environmental tone. Choo (1996) lists some of the characteristics of teachers that are positive and promote learning:

- Values learning
- Exhibits a caring relationship
- Provides learner independence
- Facilitates questioning
- Tries different approaches
- Accepts the differences among learners

Faculty are sometimes referred to as *mentor* in the teacher-student relationship. Koshenin (2004) reported on the *characteristics* of a mentoring relationship and identified five themes in the mentoring relationship that are worthy of note because they can be conceptually transferred into the classroom. They are:

- Worry about the student's adjustment
- Experience of pervasiveness of the relationship
- Feeling of mutual learning
- Worry about the learning results
- Disappointment about a lack of cooperation between the school and field (or this could be the classroom and the larger organization of academia).

Most caring teachers probably share these same concerns about how they influence student learning behaviors. The Nursing Clinical Teacher Effectiveness Inventory (NCTEI) tool that Wetherbee, Nordrum, and Giles (2008) used to evaluate clinical instructors compares credentialed and non-credentialed instructors in five general domains. The domains, rated by the students, were completed on 158 physical therapist instructors. Although the NCTEI tool was not used for nursing faculty the characteristics rated highest by students may be applicable to all clinical teaching and they include:

■ Ability
■ Interpersonal relationships
■ Personality characteristics
■ Competency
■ Evaluation strategies (Wetherbee, Nordrum, & Giles, 2008)

Kelly (2008) also studied students' perceptions of teaching effectiveness and found that there were three main important attributes for teaching effectiveness. The first of these, teacher knowledge, was rated the most important and consists of four separate domains, as listed here:

■ Teacher knowledge

    ■ As it pertains to the clinical setting
    ■ The curriculum
    ■ The learner
    ■ Teaching/learning theory

■ Feedback
■ Communication skills

Chickering and Gamson (1987) identified seven principles of good teaching practice. They define good teacher behavior as practices that:

1. Encourage contact between students and faculty,
2. Develop reciprocity and cooperation among students,
3. Encourage active learning,
4. Give prompt feedback,
5. Emphasize time on task,
6. Communicate high expectations, and
7. Respect diverse talents and ways of learning.

There are a few identifiable themes that permeate the literature when students describe a "good teacher" or "good teaching." These include the concepts of a good knowledge base, interpersonal skills, and consistent and frequent responsiveness to students. Mann (2004) provides 11 practical tips for the new college teachers designed to assist with their transition into academia. They are:

1. Do not use a red pen to correct work.
2. Provide breaks for long classes.
3. Review test answers in writing, if requested.
4. Take roll to emphasize the importance of being present.
5. Set boundaries.
6. Evaluate the advice of others and be yourself.

7. Write down your expectations.
8. Do not change textbooks during a course.
9. Attend any and all in-services you can about teaching.
10. Teach to the student level.
11. Prepare for the next year every year.

Much has been published recently about the incivility of both students and teachers in the classroom. Heinrich (2006) surveyed 261 nursing faculty and found many were willing and eager to articulate instances in which other faculty were uncivil to them. These nurses reported experiencing horizontal violence (sometimes called *lateral violence*), or "joy stealing." Some of the themes related to this phenomenon and identified in the article were:

- They were set up by administration or colleagues to fail because they were not provided with the appropriate resources.
- Administration or colleagues devalued their initiatives.
- Administration or colleagues misrepresented themselves or lied.
- Administration or colleagues shamed them by bullying them in public.
- Administrators or colleagues betrayed them.
- Administration or colleagues violated boundaries.
- Administration or colleagues divided faculty one from another.
- The "mandate game" put faculty in a win-lose situation by administration or colleagues.
- They were blamed for problems by administration or colleagues.
- They were excluded.

Student incivility will be addressed in Chapter 3. Incivility among nursing faculty is a grave concern for the profession. It is articulated here in order to make it more recognizable for faculty should they encounter uncivil treatment. Needless to say that as a profession we should have zero tolerance for incivility among ourselves, from our leaders, and from our students.

## Learning Outcomes Versus Learning Objectives

All teaching sessions begin with learning outcomes in order to frame the content or experience. Objectives and outcomes, or learning outcomes, are two terms used often in nursing education; the differences between the terms may be slight on the surface, but they depict two approaches to evaluating learning that have emerged in recent years. An objective speaks to the process; therefore, it is teacher-centric. An outcome, on the other hand, speaks to the product; thus, it is student-centric. Looking at the standard definitions of the words themselves reveals the essential difference in concepts.

1. Objective—(*noun*) something that one's efforts or actions are intended to attain or accomplish; purpose; goal; target (Dictionary.com, 2008)
2. Outcome—(*noun*) a final product or end result; consequence; issue (Diction ary.com, 2008).

An easy analogy of these terms can be related to taking a vacation. One family may plan the route and means more carefully, while another family sets their sites on the destination and the means by which they arrive there are less important.

Developing learning outcomes is done on many levels in academia. Outcomes are more general at the institutional level and more specific at the course level. Learning outcomes will vary depending on the level for which they are being developed: the entire school, a program, levels within a program, and the course-specific level.

Clinical courses can have two sets of outcomes: one set for the theory portion of the course and the second for the clinical portion. There continues to be some confusion about the difference between objectives and outcomes. Some use the terms interchangeably and argue that trying to define them is just a linguistics game, that the word *outcome* simply has been substituted for the word *objective* in order to maintain political correctness (Schwartz & Cavener, 1994). More accurately, the words represent an educational paradigm shift. The purpose for objective, or outcomes-based learning, is to provide a learner with a clear understanding of the purpose of the session, the extent of the teacher's expectations, and the extent to which a student's changed behavior demonstrates that learning has taken place (Rankin & Stalings, 2001). Objectives, or outcomes-based learning, frames the teaching and learning process that is to take place; the process is an important part of the syllabus and curriculum (DeYoung, 2003).

## Tyler's Work on Objectives

Historically, education has used objectives for student learning since Tyler's landmark book *Basic Principles of Curriculum and Instruction* (1949) encouraged educators to develop behavioral objectives to organize their teaching. Therefore, objectives are part of the behavioral paradigm. Educators adopted objective writing skills and began to use objectives to guide classroom teaching. In order to standardize the format of objectives, educators have incorporated the action verbs outlined in Bloom's Taxonomy.

## Bloom's Taxonomy

Bloom's *Taxonomy of Educational Objectives* (1956) describes an end behavior (see Table 2.8). The taxonomy uses "behavioral terms" to divide learning into leveled achievement, from knowledge acquisition to the synthesization of new ideas. Behavioral terms were further categorized into domains of cognitive, psychomotor, and affective ability to underscore the presence of the art, the science, and the practice of learning or, for our purposes, nursing. Bloom's work provided a standard method to use when evaluating and measuring learning (Novotny & Griffin, 2006).

## Gagne's Work on Objectives

Gagne (1970) reinforced the need for objectives by stating that objectives are the second event in the nine steps to instruction (please refer to Table 2.1). He

| Table 2.8 | Bloom's Taxonomy | |
|---|---|---|
| **Level** | **Concept** | **Verbs Used in Writing Objectives and Learning Outcomes** |
| Synthesis (Creating) | Explanation, comparison, illustration | Arrange, assemble, collect, compose, construct, create, design, develop, formulate, manage, organize, plan, prepare, propose, set up, write<br>Pinch (1995) has further defined the concept of synthesis as a process that includes the formation of a new product and is also language used to critically appraise literature in the profession (see evidence-based education section) |
| Evaluation (Evaluating) | Memory, repetition, description | Appraise, argue, assess, attach, choose, compare, defend, estimate, judge, predict, rate, core, select, support, value, evaluate |
| Analysis (Analyzing) | Solution, application | Analyze, appraise, calculate, categorize, compare, contrast, criticize, differentiate, discriminate, distinguish, examine, experiment, question, test |
| Application (Applying) | Induction deduction, logical order | Apply, choose, demonstrate, dramatize, employ, illustrate, interpret, operate, practice, schedule, sketch, solve, use, write |
| Comprehension (Understanding) | Productive thinking, novelty | Classify, describe, discuss, explain, express, identify, indicate, locate, recognize, report, restate, review, select, translate |
| Knowledge (Remembering) | Judgment, selection | Arrange, define, duplicate, label, list, memorize, name, order, recognize, relate, recall, repeat, reproduce, state. |

From *Taxonomy of Educational Objectives*, by B. Bloom, M. Englehart, E. Furst, W. Hill, and D. Drathwohl, 1956. New York: Longmans, Green and "The Questioning Skills of Nursing Instructors," by J. Craig, 1981. *Journal of Nursing Education, 20*(5), 18–23.

characterized objectives as a step useful to inform a learner of what is to be achieved. Using objectives served to organize the teaching and learning process while the discipline of nursing was in its growing stage of intense curriculum development (Parker, 2005).

## Paradigm Shift

Changing from objectives to outcomes is truly more of a conceptual change than an operational change. Some nurse educators have simply switched words, but not their thought processes. Others believe that neither objectives nor outcomes give us the freedom needed to encourage students to think critically (Bevis & Watson, 1989; Diekelmann, 1997). Diekelmann (1997), Bevis and Watson (1989), and others have rightfully questioned the use of objectives within today's postmodern educational environment. They understand that all learning is not displayed in behavior and that, by predetermining objectives or outcomes, we may be squelching the depth and breath of students' learning experiences. It is difficult at best to package the human intellect into a modifiable mold for convenience of grouping, evaluating, and justifying what is being taught or presented and what a learner carries forth from the experience.

## Distinguishing Between Learning Objectives and Learning Outcomes

Dr. Diane Billings stated it well when she wrote, "Outcome statements should be written to emphasize what is to be accomplished" (Billings & Halstead, 2005, p. 182). The formula for writing learning outcomes is depicted graphically in Table 2.9. With this in mind, it is important to remember that objectives can be written for curriculums, different levels of students studying within the curriculum, specific courses, or even specific class sessions.

- Using objectives was a good way to organize the teaching/learning *process* while the discipline of nursing was in its growing stage of intense curriculum development (Parker, 2005).
- Using outcomes has now become more important, and nursing education has adopted the use of "expected outcomes." Unlike objective-based learning, the process is no longer the priority in the learning. Rather, with outcome-based learning, the most important priority is to achieve the expected outcome explained in terms of *what the student will cognitively acquire by the end of the experience.*
- "Outcome statements should be written to emphasize what is to be accomplished" (Billings & Halstead, 2005, p. 182).
- Both objectives and outcomes use behavioral terms and the principles set forth by Tyler and Bloom.
- Because most educational institutions still describe learning in terms of outcomes, the formula to write them is depicted in Table 2.9.

## Developing a Lesson Plan

Lesson plans are not often spoken about in higher education to the same extent they are in primary education. In higher education, lesson plans are often simply a chart showing what learning the teacher expects to facilitate during a specific time period and how that learning facilitation is going to be accomplished. Saunders (2003) states that, "Lesson plans are beneficial because they help teachers articulate and confirm achievement of expected educational outcomes, create a historical record about the class or program, and provide a means of communicating with others" (p. 70).

| Table 2.9 | Parts of Writing a Learning Objective | | | | | |
|---|---|---|---|---|---|---|
| Antecedent | Learner | Verb Describing Behavior | Content | Context | Criteria |
| By the end of this session | the nursing student will | Demonstrate | Sterile gloving | In clinical settings | 100% of the time |

Saunders (2003) states the three goals of lesson plans:

- To ensure that educational goals are met.
- To provide a historical record of educational experiences and provide information for credentialing.
- To communicate with others about what learning is being facilitated. This may be helpful for curriculum development to assess how a specific topic is covered. In a tightly integrated curriculum, for example, faculty may share lesson plans to ensure that gaps or overlaps in content are avoided.
- An example of a teaching plan is shown in Exhibit 2.3.

## Critical Thinking

Critical thinking as the educational concept that we understand today can be traced back to 1941, when Glaser defined composites of knowledge. Other historical developments about the concept of critical thinking are as follows.

- In 1970, Perry (Nilson, 2003) expanded this by describing three distinct levels of critical thinking: dualism, relativism, and commitment.

| Exhibit 2.3 | Teaching Plan Example | | | | | | |
|---|---|---|---|---|---|---|---|
| Learning Outcomes | Related Course Objectives | Content Outline | Time | Assignment | Teaching Strategy | Equipment Needed | Evaluation |
| | | | | | | | |

Adapted from "In Control of the Lesson Plan," by S. Brink, 2008. *Los Angeles Times* (Southern California Edition), May 26, F5, p. 1.

At the NLN Summit for Nursing Education, Wilkenson and Mission (2008) presented activities that promote learners critical thinking by using:

- Lectures
- Worksheets
- Discussions
- Handouts

- In 1989, the NLN recognized the inclusion of critical thinking as a specific criterion for the accreditation of nursing programs.
- Miller and Malcolm (1990) adapted Glaser's definition into a model for critical thinking and advised educators to pay closer attention to students' mental processes.

In the early days of concept development, educators were concerned with finding an appropriate definition for critical thinking in order to evaluate its development within students. The word "critical" comes from the Greek language and means to question, discern, judge, choose, and evaluate (Jones & Brown, 1993). Other definitions of critical thinking are listed in Table 2.10.

## Evidence-Based Education

Klein and Patterson (2008) surveyed 90 faculty members from 89 different educational institutions and reached the following results about nursing education:

- 78% of faculty use lectures
- 74% use interactive strategies
- 71% use case studies
- 89% use ideas from conferences and educational articles
- Fewer than 50% felt prepared to use evidence-based education
- 22% use integrative reviews
- 22% use expert opinions

DiVito-Thomas (2005) emphasizes the importance of critical thinking by stating, "thinking critically like a nurse is becoming a benchmark of professional competence and student performance" (p. 133).

- DiVito-Thomas' qualitative study of students' perceptions of which learning techniques fostered critical thinking revealed that the most prominent theme was "more clinical time" (2005, p. 135).
- Other activities identified in the study as methods that enhance critical thinking included concept mapping, student-teacher dialogue, and case studies. This underscores the importance of facilitating critical thinking in nursing students.

Scheffer and Rubenfield (2000) developed a consensus statement describing the attributes of critical thinking that is useful for nursing education because it acknowledges the multifaceted characteristics of metacognitive skills. They are:

| Table 2.10 | Selected Definitions of Critical Thinking |
|---|---|
| **Author** | **Description of Critical Thinking** |
| Watson and Glaser (1964): (Watson-Glaser Critical Thinking Appraisal, WGCTA®, and WGCTA & Logo are trademarks of Harcourt Assessment, Inc.) | A composite of attitudes, knowledge, and skills, including: 1. Attitudes of inquiry that involve an ability to recognize the existence of problems and an acceptance of the general need for evidence in support of what is asserted to be true. 2. Knowledge of the nature of valid inferences, abstractions, and generalizations in which the weight or accuracy of different kinds of evidence are logically determined. 3. Skills in employing and applying the above attitudes and knowledge. |
| Facione, Facione, and Sanchez (1994) | Critical thinking in the process of purposeful, self-regulating judgment. |
| Paul and Elder (2007) | Attitudes are central, rather than peripheral, to critical thinking as is independence, confidence, and responsibility. These are needed to arrive at one's own judgment. |
| Bandman and Bandman (1995) | Critical thinking as the rational examination of ideas, inferences, assumptions, principles, arguments, conclusions, issues, statements, beliefs, and actions. It covers scientific reasoning and includes the nursing process, decision making, and reasoning in controversial issues. It also includes deductive, inductive, informal and practical reasoning. |

- Perseverance
- Open-mindedness
- Flexibility
- Confidence
- Creativity
- Inquisitiveness
- Reflection
- Intellectual integrity
- Intuition
- Contextual insight
- Perspective
- Information seeking
- Transformative knowledge
- Applying standards
- Logical reasoning

- Discriminating
- Analyzing

When developing the California Critical Thinking Disposition Inventory, Facione, Facione, and Sanchez (1994) provided attributes or dispositions of people who think critically. The attributes they identified include:

- Inquisitiveness
- Open mindedness
- Systematic or focused inquiry
- Analytical thinking
- Truth seeking
- Self-confidence
- Maturity

Nurse educators can *role model critical thinking* and *create opportunities for learners to develop their own critical thinking skills* by asking higher level questions and "thinking out loud," or dialoguing, about an issue from different perspectives in order to synthesize a solution.

Walker (2003) reviewed some of the teaching strategies that enhance critical thinking, and suggests that they include:

- Questioning that promotes the evaluation and synthesis of facts
- Classroom discussions and debates with open negotiation
- Short, focused writing assignments, such as:
    - "Summarize five major points in a chapter."
    - "Discuss the essence of the chapter using a metaphor."
    - "Explain the chapter to your neighbor who has a high school education."
    - "How does the chapter affect your life, personally or professionally?"

## Metacognition

Metacognition is a higher order cognitive process. Metacognitive abilities enable students to be successful learners.

- Metacognition can best be explained as the processes that are needed to organize cognitive thinking on an executive level in order for learning to take place (August-Brady, 2005; Staib, 2003; Turner, 2005).
- Metacognition includes self-direction and reflective learning and also encompasses the approach one takes to learning (Franek, Martin, & Wilkerson, 2008).
- Some studies link metacognition to intelligence, while others link it to decision-making (Livingston, 1997).
- Koriat (2008) studied how people perceive and learn in relation to memory and used an acronym, Easily Learned, Easily Remembered (ELER), to explain the study results, which found that cues that are simpler and more familiar are recalled with greater ease.

- Doherty (2005) studied the relationship of self-efficacy and metacognition as predictors of perceived decision-making in nursing students and found that metacognition explained 23% of the variances in decision making.

# Role Modeling

Positive role modeling and critical thinking appear to be related concepts in nursing education. Myrick and Yonge (2002) studied preceptor behavior ($n = 6$) through a grounded theory approach and found that new graduates' critical thinking benefited from the following positive preceptor behaviors: role modeling, facilitation, guidance, and prioritization

- Besides prompting student critical thinking with positive faculty role models, Nelms, Jones, and Gray (1993) studied role-modeling's effect on caring in nursing ($N = 137$) and found that faculty who role modeled caring promoted caring behavior in their students.
- Many times, role-modeling becomes synonymous with preceptor ability within the clinical area.
- Role-modeling in the classroom is less studied, although it has been applied to the success of minority students. Newton (2008) has addressed role-modeling in relation to publications and the dissemination of nursing knowledge.

# Evidence-Based Education (EBE)

The foundations of EBE are analogous to the evidence-based practice (EBP) literature in nursing science. One of the important points for nurse educators to keep in mind is the synthesis of evidence in an organized framework that can be appraised in order to draw a conclusion or develop an opinion that is grounded and derived from logical, common ideas in the literature (Pinch, 1995). Emerson and Records (2008) call on all nurse educators to take a part in developing EBE and to identify catalysts for change to promote EBE:

- Societal mandates insists on quality education mandated through accrediting and governmental agencies with an ever-increasing emphasis on public safety.
- In terms of priorities for funding, there has been a lack of academic recognition of the value of nursing education research in promotion and tenure criteria.
- The Core Competencies of Nurse Educators was developed by The National League for Nursing (NLN, 2005) and has identified competencies related to scholarship and the practice of evidence-based teaching as listed here.
  - Competency One addresses the expectation that nurse educators will create environments for facilitating student learning and the

achievement of desired cognitive, affective, and psychomotor outcomes. This competency is applicable across didactic, clinical, and laboratory settings. To facilitate learning effectively, nurse educators must ground the choice of teaching strategies in educational theory and evidence-based teaching practices.

- Competency Three concerns assessment and evaluation strategies used by nurse educators.

  - This competency charges faculty with the responsibility of using a variety of strategies to assess and evaluate student learning in the classroom, laboratory, and clinical settings, as well as in all domains of learning.
  - To use assessment and evaluation strategies effectively, nurse educators must use existing literature to develop evidence-based assessment and evaluation approaches and implement evidence-based assessment and evaluation strategies that are appropriate for learners and the learning goals.
  - Nurse educators are also charged with demonstrating skill in the design and implementation of assessment tools related to clinical practice.

- Competency Seven requires nurse educators to acknowledge scholarship as an integral component of their faculty role and to acknowledge teaching as a scholarly activity. To engage effectively in scholarship, nurse educators exhibit a spirit of inquiry about teaching and learning, student development, evaluation methods, and other aspects of the role; design and implement scholarly activities in an established area of expertise; disseminate nursing and teaching knowledge to a variety of audiences through various means; demonstrate skill in proposal writing for initiatives that include, but are not limited to, research, resource acquisition, program development, and policy development; and demonstrate qualities of a scholar, including integrity, courage, perseverance, vitality, and creativity (NLN, 2005).

- Fostering risk taking and replacing older pedagogies with active learning strategies
- Re-envisioning promotion and tenure (Please see Chapter 8.)
- Fulfilling the university mission

Ferguson and Day (2005) states that nursing education still needs much more quantitative and qualitative research to improve the science of nursing education. EBE is based on four elements:

- Evidence—both quantitative and qualitative
- Professional judgment—nurse educators' decision-making ability
- Values of students as clients—using judgment appropriately by getting to know the students
- Resource issues—money, time, and space

# Teaching Strategies

Teaching strategies are the way in which a teacher presents or facilitates the presentation of course content. Teaching strategies encompass endless ways of delivery, but can be categorized into subtopics. These are passive and active teaching strategies.

■ Passive teaching strategies do not involve the learner, but are still in use because they may be an effective mode for delivering large amounts of content.
■ Active teaching strategies are the ones that make a classroom come alive, and engage the learner.
■ Most every teacher uses a combination of passive (such as lecture) and active (such as group projects) teaching strategies.

## Passive Strategies

Lecturing is the most commonly used passive teaching strategy. It has the advantage of allowing a teacher to cover a large amount of material in a relatively short amount of time.

■ Lectures are rarely used in their pure form, with a teacher informing students by just speaking to them.
■ Lectures are most often used with audio or visual supplements.
■ One of the most common visual tools is Microsoft's PowerPoint® presentation software. PowerPoint can be used effectively with graphics, pictures, sounds, and new clicker technology to liven up a lecture.
■ Many other strategies can also be interspersed within a lecture to create a more active environment, such as games, discussion, or group activity (Oermann, 2004).

Diekelmann (1997) challenges schools to foster student-faculty partnerships "to overcome barriers to learning such as: passive instruction, teacher-talk, student silence, and the denial of subjects in the curriculum that are important to students" (p. 147).

In 1984, Campsey wrote an article about lecturing guidelines that is still valuable today if lecture is used to some extent in the classroom. These guidelines include:

■ Be aware that mild speaking anxiety is normal.
■ Be as prepared as possible.
■ Never memorize.
■ Never read word for word.
■ Rehearse.
■ Think positively.
■ If possible, lecture on content that you know well.
■ Show enthusiasm for the subject.
■ Have only two or three learning objectives per hour.

- Assess the room.
- Use teaching aides (you may know these as "active learning strategies").
- Use plain language whenever possible. (This is important, with today's classes that may include any number of students who learned English as a second, or even third, language.)
- Do not be authoritarian.
- Watch non-verbal clues.

In 1989, Cooper added some more criteria to the list of lecturing do's and don'ts, including:

- Do use examples, these are the basis for case studies.
- Do evaluate your presentation after it ends to make immediate adjustments for next time.
- Don't hurry.
- Don't use a lecture if another approach is appropriate.

Darbyshire (1995) called for schools to consider a nursing humanities course in which nursing students could gain meaning through works of literature, such as William Stryron's *Darkness Visible*. Using literary works as teaching tools in nursing needs further research.

Creative teaching enhances critical thinking and has been studied as a method for developing new or novel ideas. Teachers who employ creative thinking use techniques such as overdramatization, humor, and risk taking in the classroom (Kalischuk & Thorpe, 2002). (For further information on teaching strategies, please see Chapter 7.)

## PowerPoint®

PowerPoint is as ubiquitous today as the use of transparencies and slide shows were in the past, but it features many more designs, transitions, and capabilities. Educational literature warns about the poor use of PowerPoint. Abe (2008) encourages instructors to have a neutral person evaluate their PowerPoint presentations for criteria such as:

- Flow of ideas
- Visual appeal
- Wordiness
- Readability
- Distracting backgrounds
- Font size
- Image clarity
- Entertainment factor

## Active Strategies

Most educators stress the importance of providing frequent active learning strategies, including breaks and short physical exercise activities, interspersed throughout a presentation in order to hold learners' interest. Bremner et al. (2008) reinforces that exercise increases oxygen flow and improves cognition;

therefore, short, active breaks enhance the classroom learning experience. Table 2.11 presents a variety of passive and active teaching strategies

## Active Learning

Active learning is a common term in nursing education. In the past, teachers were expected to "pour" knowledge into their students as if they were some type of container that could be filled with facts (Luse, 2002).

- We now know that learning is a social activity that is best accomplished in an interactive environment (Vygotsky, 1978).
- Active learning assists students to not only take part in their own learning, but also challenges them to take responsibility for their learning (Billmeyer & Barton, 1998).

## Cooperative/Collaborative Learning Techniques

- These techniques support active learning using a peer-centered approach.
- This is an overall framework that supports many kinds of active learning techniques with a special focus on group engagement, such as learning circles and project-based learning (Treschuk, 2008).

## Self-Learning

Self-learning is another term often heard in nursing education.

- Hao and Meng (2006) explain the concept well by stating, "Self-learning is completely student-centered. Learners decide their learning goals, choose the contents which they want to learn, and arrange the sequences of their learning, etc" (p. 116).

## Classroom Techniques

- Zsohar and Smith (2006) have composed a list of the "top 10 don'ts" for classroom teaching. (For more on oral questioning in the classroom, see Exhibit 2.4):

1. Don't be late for class.
2. Don't pretend knowledge.
3. Don't read or repeat information that is easily accessible to the learner.
4. Don't bring personal baggage into class.
5. Don't come unprepared with excuses for a lack of preparation.
6. Don't be confrontational.
7. Don't interrupt.
8. Don't devalue the content taught by colleagues.
9. Don't be inconsistent with expectations.
10. Don't forget to be passionate about teaching.

| Table 2.11 | Teaching Strategies | | |
| --- | --- | --- | --- |
| Strategy | Description | Advantage | Disadvantage |
| Passive Strategies | | | |
| Demonstration | Models a skill or behavior | Effective for learning in the psychomotor domain. Actively engages the learner. Visually shows a process that often aids in retention (Bastable, 2007; Billings & Halstead, 2005) | High faculty workload. Requires small groups and adequate time. Equipment may be costly to purchase and replace. |
| Lecture | Highly-structured teacher presentation, often accompanied by a PowerPoint presentation and handouts. It is one of the oldest and most often used approaches to teaching. | Cost-effective. Targets large groups. Better for lower levels of cognitive activity (Bastable, 2007; Billings & Halstead, 2005) | Decreases student involvement. Lengthy preparation time for faculty. Not individualized. |
| Role modeling | Models a skill or behavior | Helps with socialization | Requires rapport |
| Active Learning Strategies | | | |
| Algorithms | Algorithms are maps that break down decision-making about clinical issues into step-by-step procedures that lead learners to yes or no answers. | Demonstrates to the learner exactly what is important to consider. Saves explanation time. | Developing is time consuming (Rowles & Brigham, 2005). |
| Case studies | Uses a scenario about a patient for analysis and decision-making (Joel, 2007). One method uses the framework of identifying focal, contextual, and residual stimuli in the case (DeSanto-Madeya, 2007). | Effective and promotes critical thinking. | Takes time to develop cases. |

*(Continued)*

| Table 2.11 | Teaching Strategies (Continued) | | |
|---|---|---|---|
| Concept (cognitive) mapping | Visual representation to illustrate relationships between concepts (Joel, 2007). Knowledge is arranged hierarchically (All & Havens, 1997). | Promotes critical thinking by using prior knowledge to connect new concepts. | Time consuming for faculty. |
| Clinical conferences | Using questioning techniques to elicit higher cognitive levels and more student dialogue. | Rossignol (2000) found a direct link between the cognitive level of the questioning and the cognitive discourse of the students. | Students are tired after the clinical day. Some instructors do post conference in a discussion board format. |
| Collaborative learning | Teams of learners work on assignments and assume responsibility for group learning outcomes. | Promotes active and reflective learning. Encourages teamwork. Provides an opportunity for students to become accountable for their own work. | Students may resist frequent use of group assignments. It is possible that all students will not participate equally. |
| Debate | The process of inquiry or reasoned judgment on a proposition aimed at demonstrating the truth or falsehood of something; involves the construction of logical arguments and oral defense of a proposition. | Develops analytical skills. Develops students' ability to recognize complexities in many health care issues. Broadens views of controversial topics. Develops communication skills. | Requires a fairly high level of knowledge about subject on the parts of both those presenting the debate and the audience. May require teaching students the art of debate. Requires increased student preparation. Can cause anxiety and conflict for students because of the confrontational nature of debate. |

*(Continued)*

| Table 2.11 | Teaching Strategies (Continued) | | |
|---|---|---|---|
| **Strategy** | **Description** | **Advantage** | **Disadvantage** |
| Discussions | A way to solve problems as a group. Usually the teacher gives the students information to prepare prior to the class time. The time in class is used to engage in clarification information and concepts. This is very effective for smaller groups but it does take time (DeYoung, 2003). | One of the most effective strategies for active learning because it allows learners to think critically about the topic being discussed (Johnson & Mighten, 2005). | May not engage students who are introverts. |
| Games | Can increase problem solving ability and increase learning retention (Royse & Newton, 2007). One of the most effective type of games is Jeopardy | Promotes active, engaged learning. | Games take time to make and implement. |
| Group discussion | Learners exchange information, feelings, and opinions with one another and the teacher (Bastable, 2007; Billings & Halstead, 2005). | Enhances learning in both the affective and cognitive domains. Stimulates learners to share and think about issues and problems. Fosters peer support. | One or more class members may dominate the discussion. Easy to digress from the topic. More time consuming to transmit knowledge. Requires teacher's presence to keep students focused on topic at hand. |
| Humor | Using the incongruencies in life with words or art work is commonly used to stimulate learning (Starr, 2009) | Stimulates thought | Must be politically correct to avoid insulting any group. There needs to be more research about its effect (Starr, 2009). |

*(Continued)*

| Table 2.11 | Teaching Strategies (Continued) | | |
|---|---|---|---|
| Imagery/Art | Art has been used to increase students' observational and communication skills (Nordon, 2005). | Stimulates cognitive thinking and teamwork through discussion. | Time considerations |
| Jigsaw activity | Different students are assigned components of a larger learning module and they all place the pieces together. | Suggested as an online activity, but can be adapted for in-class use (Beitz & Snarponis, 2006) | Time considerations |
| One-to-one instruction | Delivers instruction that is designed to meet the needs of one learner | Pace and content can be individualized. Good for teaching behavior in all three domains. Good for students with learning disabilities. Provides immediate feedback (Bastable, 2007; Billings & Halstead, 2005). | The learner is isolated from others who have similar needs. Learners cannot share information, ideas, or feelings with others. Learners may feel anxious or overwhelmed if the teacher provides much content. |
| Problem-based learning | Uses a group method for learning. It promotes cooperation in learning. A problem or case is given to the group and the learners take responsibility to understand the presented material. The teacher's role is one of facilitator or tutor. The role of the tutor is reportedly of extreme importance in the success of PBL (Mete & Sari, 2008) It originated at the McMaster Medical School in the late 1960s (Jones & Sheppard, 2008). | Produces effective self-learning skills and may be more enjoyable for the student (Beers & Bowden, 2005). | Effectiveness questioned (Beers & Bowden, 2005) and may be more difficult with large groups of students. |

*(Continued)*

| Table 2.11 | Teaching Strategies (Continued) | | |
|---|---|---|---|
| **Strategy** | **Description** | **Advantage** | **Disadvantage** |
| Reflection journaling | Used many times for gaining insight into clinical experiences. Assists learning in the cognitive and affective domains. Can be prompted by a specific, open-ended question or free style (Joel, 2007). | Encourages self-reflection and assists in critical thinking. | May place faculty in an awkward ethical position if students reveal personal issues. |
| Return demonstration | The learner attempts to perform a task with cues from the teacher, as needed (Bastable, 2007; Billings & Halstead, 2005) | Effective for learning in the psychomotor domain. Actively engages the learner. Repetition increases confidence, competence, and skill retention. | Requires time for teaching as well as learning. Groups must be small. Involves costly equipment and space. |
| Role-playing | Unscripted role-playing assists students to develop understanding of other people's and patients' situations (Joel, 2007). | Encourages the student to empathize in the role. | May be difficult or distressing for students who are reticent. |
| Seminar | A meeting for an exchange of ideas in some area (Bastable, 2007; Billings & Halstead, 2005) | Collaborative, cooperative learning, peer sharing, and dialogue facilitate comprehension and practical application of concepts. Active student engagement with content. | Requires that students possess adequate knowledge for active discussion and comprehension. May require greater amount of student preparation time. Students will require instruction on how to prepare. |

*(Continued)*

| Table 2.11 | Teaching Strategies (Continued) | | |
|---|---|---|---|
| Student-generated quizzes and case studies | Students have to extract material based on the required readings. | Active learning strategies that assists the student to share their work and think on a different level. (Beitz & Snarponis, 2006) | Time and evaluation considerations. |
| Storytelling (narrative) | Powerful communication tool and can be done in a variety of formats, such as legends, poems, myths, novels, films, fairy tales, fables or plays (Davidhizar & Lonser, 2003). | Maintain cultural heritage. Has personal appeal to students. | Time considerations. Short stories work well with lectures. |
| Top ten list | Students prioritize topics from their reading in a list format | Helps students to organize, prioritize, and compare their results with others (Beitz & Snarponis, 2006) | May differ from student to student. |
| Tutorials self-learning packets | Self-learning packets are currently used in electronic, hypertext form (Johnson & Mighten, 2005). | Lays out all the information for the class on disk and allows students to work at their own pace. | May not be effective for students who tend to procrastinate. |
| Questioning for critical thinking (Socratic) | "Questioning helps students to think critically when making clinical decisions" (Wink, 1993, p. 11). Questions may include: Formulate the question clearly (frame them in the context of what is being discussed). Remember to give the student time to formulate the answer—"three-second rule." | Questioning has long been used (from the time of Socrates) as a technique to encourage critical thinking. | Can be intimidating to the student if not done in an emancipatory learning environment. |

*(Continued)*

| Table 2.11 | Teaching Strategies (Continued) | | |
|---|---|---|---|
| Strategy | Description | Advantage | Disadvantage |
| | Ask follow-up questions such as Why? Do you agree or disagree? Can you elaborate on that? House, Chassie, and Spohn (1999) describe questions as falling into one of two categories:<br>■ Convergent, those that are low level and elicit factual answers<br>■ Divergent, higher level and provoke student thinking. | | |
| Unfolding case studies | Unfolding case studies differ from traditional case studies because they evolve over time (Karani, Leipzig, Callahan, & Thomas, 2004). They help students to "develop skills they need to analyze, organize and prioritize in novel situations" (Batscha & Moloney, 2005, p. 387). They more closely mimic real-life situations in nursing and are a *situational mental model* that assists students to problem solve, actively engage, and use critical thinking techniques (Azzarello & Wood, 2006). | Assists students to interpose some "real life" scenarios with their theoretical learning. | They take time to develop and students work through them at different rates. |
| Value clarification | Value clarification exercises assist students as they sort out what they value so they can better understand how their values may be affecting patient care and | These exercises assist students to reflect and to understand each other. | These exercises take time and facilitation. |

*(Continued )*

| Table 2.11 | Teaching Strategies (Continued) | | |
|---|---|---|---|
| | decision-making. There are many kinds of value clarification exercises, including: ordering, prizing, and affirming beliefs (Wittmann-Price, 2007). | | |
| Vignettes | Short stories or case studies often left incomplete to allow room for discussion (Kish, 2007). | Encourage active adult learning strategies in students. | May be difficult for educators who are not clinically active in the field. |
| Warm-up/ start up exercises | Activities to check reading assignments at the beginning of class. They can count for a partial grade. | Encourages students to read prior to class. | Takes class time. |

| Exhibit 2.4 | Benefits of Oral Questioning |
|---|---|

Seven Key Benefits of Oral Questioning:

1.  Increases motivation and participation
2.  Helps monitor the learners' acquisition of knowledge and understanding
3.  Promotes higher cognition
4.  Assesses learners' progress
5.  Facilitates classroom management
6.  Encourages learners to ask and to answer questions
7.  Promotes dialogue/interaction/debate between and among teacher and students (Ralph, 2000)

# Evidence-Based Education

Jones and Sheppard (2008) used a randomized control trial of students ($N = 60$) in an Associate degree program to test problem-based learning (PBL). The intervention group scored higher on post-test critical thinking and communication evaluation.

## Reflective Education

- In 1983, Schon published his landmark book, *The Reflective Practitioner: How Professionals Think in Action,* and called upon educators to develop themselves as reflective practitioners in order to gain competence in their individual practices.

- Boud et al. (1985) defined reflection as "an important human activity in which people recapture their experience, think about it, mull it over, and evaluate it" (p. 19).

- Reflection is a technique that encourages critical thought, either with oneself (self-dialogue) or another individual or group (dialogue) (Shor, 1992).

- Reflection is a self-analytical process that surfaces contradictions between what one intends to achieve in any given situation and the way one is behaving (Johns, 1999), and considers both the person and the situation (Penney & Warelow, 1999).

## Evidence-Based Education

Reflection is said to create independence from the teacher. Lowe and Kerr (1998) divided students into two groups: one that was exposed to reflective learning techniques and one that underwent conventional learning ($N = 46$). They found the outcome measure (testing knowledge, comprehension, and application) of learning was not significantly different between groups, therefore reflective techniques were able to promote the intended outcome just as well as conventional techniques.

### Journaling

Nurse educators have historically encouraged reflective thinking techniques via journaling. Part of the initiative started when Allen, Bowers, and Diekelmann (1989) reconceptualized writing by using it as a learning strategy, not just as a recitation one.

- Journaling is an excellent self-analysis technique for both students and teachers.

- Many nurse educators use the technique after a clinical day in a free flow attempt to assist students to uncover what affective behaviors they can identify as assess, and to highlight those behaviors that may be deficits.

- Others pose reflective questions to students, such as "What was the one thing (incident or patient) that affected you most today?" or "What was the best thing that happened to you today?"

- Usually questions like these are followed up with questions such as, "What one thing would you do differently if you were in that situation again?"
- Several issues must be considered when asking students to journal:
  - Journals are a self-disclosing process that can elicit sensitive information.
  - What one does with information revealed during journaling may become an ethical issue; little has been written about this particular dilemma in nursing education.

### Journaling as a Mentoring Model

- Bilinski (2002) describes the teacher-student-journaling relationship as a mentoring model.
- The mentored journal establishes a collaborative relationship that increases critical thinking.
- The faculty member supports the student's journaling and facilitates the student to find deeper meanings in the experiences they have recorded.

Riley-Doucet and Wilson (1997) describe a three-step process for reflective journaling:

- *Critical appraisal* is journaling done by a student in free form to drill down to the meaning of the clinical experience.
- *Peer group discussion* shares questions that the students might have become aware of during the journaling process.
- *Self-awareness* or *self evaluation* is the last step and relates journaling to clinical objectives for evaluative purposes.

## Classroom Management

The underpinning of positive classroom management is respect for the students. Once an atmosphere of trust and respect is established, there should be very few classroom management issues. Classroom management is also very different today when compared to the past, due to large class sizes and the advent of new technologies. Both of these issues have implications for classroom management. According to Mulligan (2007), there are four pillars of classroom management:

- Pillar 1: Instructional strategies that motivate and keep students interested and engaged.
- Pillar 2: Uses instructional time wisely and is a proactive approach to teaching; charges the students to be accountable for their learning.
- Pillar 3: Social behaviors that need attention and correcting.
- Pillar 4: Create a flexible environment in order to adjust to the learners' needs.

Student use of technology in the classroom has also become a concern for nurse educators. Establishing ground rules early in the course and communicating them clearly may assist to maintain classroom management.

## Closing and Not Just "Ending" a Course

*So the course is over. I enter my office, turn on the light, and begin to consider how I will facilitate closure for the next group of students. Just like caring for a patient, the process starts well before I ever meet them. (Yonge, Lee, & Luhanga, 2006, p. 151)*

# CASE STUDIES

## Case Study 2.1

Marcia is a new faculty member at a small baccalaureate school of nursing. She is full-time, tenure track, and working on her doctorate degree. Marcia is assigned a mentor and a 12-credit semester teaching load, which is normal for many institutions. She meets with her mentor who goes over her syllabus with her. The mentor asks Marcia why she has so many assignments in a clinical course. Marcia states that she believes that the students' writing skills are lacking and they need writing assignments. If you were the mentor and saw a novice place 50% of the clinical coarse grade on writing assignments, how would you handle it?

## Case Study 2.2

A seasoned faculty member has been placed in the accelerated student curriculum. There are a large number of students, and she has 10 clinical groups with seven different adjunct instructors. She uses the same syllabus as the traditional undergraduates whom she taught successfully last semester. The students have an assignment on the syllabus to pick a patient and create a complete care plan for him or her, including assessment, diagnoses, planning implementation, and evaluation format. The writing criteria state that the plan should be in APA format and approximately 10–12 pages long. The instructor gives the students a rubric to go by, and the majority of students complete the assignment on time. At the end of the semester, the educator is taken aback that the students had so many negative comments about the care plan assignment. If you were the educator, how would you alter the assignment yet still ensure that you meet the course learning outcomes of developing a plan of care for a complex client?

## Practice Questions

1. The nurse educator should expect to observe the following characteristics in the reticent student:
   A.  Inability to stay on task
   B.  Inability to contribute to a group project
   C.  Inability to control outbursts
   D.  Inability to show emotion

2. Which type of post-lesson questions should the nurse educator expect to be asked by beginning students who are visual learners when reviewing information from a tape of heart sounds?
   A.  Knowledge-based questions
   B.  Comprehension questions
   C.  Application questions
   D.  Evaluation questions

3. When assessing the capabilities of a freshman student in the lab during a simulated experience, a nurse educator should expect the student to be at which level of Bloom's Taxonomy about basic cardiac function?
   A.  Knowledge
   B.  Comprehension
   C.  Application
   D.  Evaluation

4. Which finding should the nurse educator *least* expect when assessing the learning outcomes in the current curriculum?
   A.  They are evidence-based
   B.  The process is prescribed
   C.  The outcome is clear
   D.  They are leveled

5. Which finding should a nurse educator expect when evaluating a new faculty member in the classroom?
   A.  Mild speaking anxiety
   B.  An unorganized presentation
   C.  Confidence to speak without references
   D.  Extreme speaking anxiety

6. When a nurse educator suspects a student has a learning disability, he or she should:
   A.  Test the student's IQ
   B.  Refer the student to the learning center
   C.  Provide him or her with extra time for tests
   D.  Take away some of the student's assignments

7. A nurse educator uses a tool to assess a class of students to determine the group's most prominent learning style. To elicit the information effectively, he or she should:
   A.  Ask students to work in groups
   B.  Provide students with time in class to complete the assessment

    C.  Ask students to complete the assessment at home

    D.  Tell students the scoring parameters before the tool is given

8.  When interviewing for a job, a nurse educator is asked about her education philosophy and says that she is primarily concerned with equality in the classroom. This nurse educator most likely subscribes to the philosophy of

    A.  Phenomenological

    B.  Emancipatory education

    C.  Narrative pedagogy

    D.  Constructivism

9.  At a faculty retreat a nurse educator is telling the group about her philosophy and says, "I believe in rewarding students for good behavior and doing well on tests." What philosophy is the educator a proponent of?

    A.  Realism

    B.  Essentialism

    C.  Perennialism

    D.  Behaviorism

10.  Which statement by a student should alert a nurse educator to difficulty with the material?

    A.  "I have never been given such low grades before."

    B.  "I read the book before class."

    C.  "I do extra questions every night."

    D.  "I understand the material in class, but cannot pick the right test answer."

## References

Abe, D. (2008). Teacher upgrade: PowerPoint unplugged: Presenting information and keeping your audience. *International Journal of Childbirth Education, 23*(1), 20–21.

All, A. C., & Havens, R. L. (1997). Cognitive/concept mapping: A teaching strategy for nursing. *Journal of Advanced Nursing, 25,* 1210–1219.

Allen, D., Bowers, B., & Diekelmann, N. (1989). Writing to learn: A reconceptualization of thinking and writing in the nursing curriculum. *Journal of Nursing Education, 28,* 6–11.

Arhin, A. O., & Cormiere, E. (2007). Using deconstruction to educate generation Y students. *Nursing Education, 46*(12), 562–567.

August-Brady, M. (2005). The effect of a metacognitive intervention on approach to and self-regulation of learning in baccalaureate nursing students. *Journal of Nursing Education, 44*(7), 297–304.

Azzarello, J., & Wood, D. E. (2006). Assessing dynamic mental models: Unfolding case studies. *Nurse Educator, 31*(1), 10–14.

Bandman, E. L., & Bandman, B. (1995). *Critical thinking in nursing* (2nd ed.). Norwalk, CT: Appleton & Lange.

Bandura, A. (1997). *Self-efficacy: The exercise of control.* New York: W. H. Freeman and Co.

Bastable, S. B. (2007). *Nurse as educator: Teaching and learning for nursing practice.* Boston: Jones and Bartlett Publishers.

Batscha, C., & Moloney, B. (2005). Using Powerpoint® to enhance unfolding case studies. *Journal of Nursing Education, 44*(8), 387.

Beers, G. W., & Bowden, S. (2005). The effect of teaching method on long-term knowledge retention. *Journal of Nursing Education, 44*(11), 511–514.

Beitz, J., & Snarponis, J. (2006). Strategies for online teaching and learning. *Nurse Educator, 31*(1), 20–24.

Bentley, R. (2006). Comparison of traditional and accelerated baccalaureate nursing graduates. *Nurse Educator, 31*(2), 79–83.

Berragan, L. (1998). Nursing practice draws upon several different ways of knowing. *Journal of Clinical Nursing, 7,* 209–217.

Bevis, E., & Watson, J. (1989). *Toward a caring curriculum: A new pedagogy for nursing.* New York: NLN Publications.

Bilinski, H. (2002). The mentored journal. *Nurse Educator, 27*(1), 37–41.

Billings, D., & Halstead, J. (2005). *Teaching in nursing: A guide for faculty.* St. Louis, MO: Elsevier Saunders.

Billmeyer, R., & Barton, M. L. (1998). *Teaching reading in the content areas: If not me, then who?* Aurora, CO: McREL.

Bloom, B., Englehart, M., Furst, E., Hill, W., & Drathwohl, D. (Eds.). (1956). *Taxonomy of educational objectives.* New York: Longmans, Green.

Boud, D., Keogh, R., & Walker, D. (1985). In D. Boud, R. Keogh, & D. Walker (Eds.), *Reflection: Turning experience into learning* (pp. 7–8). London: Kogan.

Bradshaw, M. J., & Nugent, K. (1997). News, notes & tips: Clinical learning experiences of non-traditional age nursing students. *Nurse Educator, 22*(6), 40, 47.

Brancato, V. (2007). Teaching for the Learner. In B. Moyer & R. A. Wittmann-Price (Eds.), *Nursing education: Foundations of practice excellence* (pp. 87–103). Philadelphia: F.A. Davis Company.

Breckinridge, D., Bower, T., Kinser, A., & Miko, C. (2008, Sept. 18). *Keywords for evidence-based teaching practice.* Paper presented at the meeting of the National League for Nursing Educational Summit, San Antonio, TX.

Bremner, M. N., Aduddell, K. F., & Amason, J. S. (2008). Evidence-based practices related to the human patient simulation and first year baccalaureate nursing students' anxiety. *Online Journal of Nursing Informatics, 12*(1), 10 pages.

Brink, S. (2008). In control of the lesson plan. *Los Angeles Times* (Southern California Edition), May 26, F5, p. 1.

Brophy, J. (1986). *On motivating students. Occasional Paper No. 101.* East Lansing, Michigan: Institute for Research on Teaching, Michigan State University.

Campsey, K. (1984). Lecturing guidelines. *The Journal of Continuing Education in Nursing, 15*(2), 68–70.

Chauvin, B. (2008, Sept. 19). *The transformation of the second-degree accelerated student.* Paper presented at the meeting of the National League for Nursing Educational Summit, San Antonio, TX.

Chickering, A. W., & Gamson, Z. F. (1987). Seven principles for good practice in undergraduate education. *The Wingspread Journal, 9*(2). Retrieved February 2007, from http://www.john sonfdn.org/Publications/ConferenceReports/SevenPrinciples

Chinn, P. (2007). Philosophical foundations for excellence in nursing. In B. Moyer & R. A. Wittmann-Price (Eds.), *Nursing education: Foundations of practice excellence* (pp.15–28). Philadelphia: F.A. Davis Company.

Choo, L. A. (1996). Reflections: learning at work. *Professional Nurse, Singapore, 23*(3), 8–11.

Cooper, S. S. (1989). Teaching tips: Some lecturing dos and don'ts. *The Journal of Continuing Education in Nursing, 20*(3), 140–141.

Cowan, D., Roberts, J., Fitzpatrick, J., While, A., & Baldwin, J. (2004). The approaches to learning of support workers employed in the care home sector: An evaluation study. *Nurse Education Today, 24,* 98–104.

Craig, J. (1981). The Questioning skills of nursing instructors. *Journal of Nursing Education, 20*(5), 18–23.

Csokasy, J. (2005). Philosophical foundations of the curriculum. In D. Billings & J. A. Halstead (Eds.), *Teaching in nursing: A guild for faculty* (pp. 125–144). St. Louis, MO: Elsevier Saunders.

Darbyshire, P. (1995). Lessons for literature: Caring, interpretation and dialogue. *Journal of Nursing Education, 34*(5), 211–216.

Davidhizar, R., & Lonser, G. (2003). Storytelling as a teaching technique. *Nurse Educator, 28*(5), 217–221.

Davis, M. (1993). The learning context: Curriculum models. *Nursing Times, 89*(40), 6–12.

DeSanto-Madeya, S. (2007). Using case studies based on a nursing conceptual model to teach medical-surgical nursing. *Nursing Science Quarterly, 20*(4), 324–329.

DeYoung, S. (2003). *Teaching strategies for nurse educators.* Upper Saddle River, NJ: Prentice Hall.

Diekelmann, N. L. (1988). Curriculum revolution: A theoretical and philosophical mandate for change. In *Curriculum revolution: Mandate for change.* New York: NLN.

Diekelmann, N. L. (1995). Reawakening thinking: Is traditional pedagogy nearing completion? *Journal of Nursing Education, 34*(5), 195–196.

Diekelmann, N. L. (1997). Creating a new pedagogy for nursing. *Journal of Nursing Education, 36*(4), 147–148.

Diekelmann, N. L., & Scheckel, M. (2004). Leaving the safe harbor of competency-based and outcomes education: Re-thinking practice education. *Journal of Nursing Education, 43*(9), 385–388.

Diseth, A. (2002). The relationship between intelligence, approaches to learning and academic achievement. *Scandinavian Journal of Educational Research, 46,* 381–394.

DiVito-Thomas, P. (2005). Nursing students stories on learning how to think like a nurse. *Nurse Educator, 30*(3), 133–136.

Doherty, T. S. (2005). *Self-efficacy and metacognition awareness as predictors of perceived decision-making in nursing students.* Unpublished manuscript, State University of New York at Albany.

Driscoll, M. P. (2000). *Psychology of learning for instruction* (2nd ed.). Needham Heights, MA: Allyn & Bacon.

Dunn, R., Dunn, K., & Price, G. (1996). *Learning style inventory.* Lawrence, KS: Price Systems.

Ellsworth, J. (1998). *Overview of Educational Philosophies.* Retrieved August 2, 2008, from http://jan.ucc.nau.edu/~jde7/ese502/assessment/lesson.html

Emerson, R. J., & Records, K. (2008). Today's challenge, tomorrow's excellence: The practice of evidence-based education. *Journal of Nursing Education, 47*(8), 359–370.

Entwistle, N. J. (1999). Approaches to studying and levels of understanding: the influences of teaching and assessment. In J. C. Smart (Ed.), *Higher education: Handbook of theory and research.* New York: Agathon Press.

Facione, N. C., Facione, P. A., & Sanchez, C. A. (1994). Critical thinking disposition as a measure of competent judgment: the development of the California Critical Disposition Inventory, *Journal of Nursing Education, 33,* 345–350.

Ferguson, L., & Day, R. (2005). Evidence-based nursing education: Myth or reality. *Journal of Nursing Education, 44*(3), 107–115.

Filipczak, B. (1995). Out of the can: How to customize off the shelf education. *Education, 32,* 51–57.

Fleming, N. (2009). VARK: A guide to learning style. Retrieved March 29, 2009, from http://www.vark-learn.com/english/index.asp

Franek, T. B., Martin, M., & Wilkerson, G. B. (2008). Metacognition in athletic training education. *Athletic Therapy Today, 13*(4), 2–4.

Freire, P. (1970). *Pedagogy of the oppressed.* New York: Continuum Publishing Company.

Freshman, B., & Rubino, L. (2002). Emotional intelligence: A care competency for health care administrators. *Health Care Management, 21*(4), 1–9.

Gagne, R. (1970). *The conditions of learning* (2nd ed.). New York: Holt, Rinehart and Winston.

Glaser, E. M. (1941). *An experiment in the development of critical thinking,* New York: Teacher's College, Columbia University.

Grady, C. (2008, Sept. 19). *Faculty notions of caring in male nursing students.* Paper presented at the meeting of the National League for Nursing Educational Summit, San Antonio, TX.

Grady, C., Stewardson, G., & Hall, J. (2008). Faculty notions regarding caring in male nursing students. *Journal of Nursing Education, 47*(7), 314–223.

Grasha, A. (1996). *Teaching with Style.* Pittsburgh, PA: Alliance Publishers.

Hao, X., & Meng, X. (2006). The research as a kind of knowledge network for self-learning. *Edutainment, 3942,* 116–123.

Heinrich, K. (2006). Joy stealing: 10 mean games faculty play and how to stop the gaming, *Nurse Educator, 32*(1), 34–38.

Hezekiah, J. (1993). Feminist pedagogy: A framework for nursing education? *Journal of Nursing Education, 32*(2), 53–57.

Honey, P., & Mumford, A. (2006). *What kind of learner are you?* London: Campaign for Learning.

House, B. M., Chassie, M. B., & Spohn, B. B. (1999). Questioning: An essential ingredient in effective teaching. *The Journal of Continuing Education in Nursing, 21*(5), 196–201.

Humphreys, A., Thompson, N., & Miner, K. (1998). Assessment of breastfeeding intention using the transtheoretical model and the theory of reasoned action. *Health Education Research Theory and Practice, 13,* 331–341.

Joel, L. (2007). Instructional Methods. In B. Moyer & R. A. Wittmann-Price (Eds.), *Nursing education: Foundations of practice excellence* (pp. 183–205). Philadelphia: F.A. Davis Company.

Johns, C. (1999). Reflection as empowerment? *Nursing Inquiry, 6,* 241–249.

Johnson, J. P., & Mighten, A. (2005). A comparison of teaching strategies: Lecture notes combined with structured group discussion versus lecture only. *Journal of Nursing Education, 44*(7), 319–322.

Johnson, S. A., & Romanello, M. L. (2005). Generational diversity: Teaching and learning approaches. *Nurse Educator, 30*(5), 212–216.

Jones, S. A., & Brown, L. N. (1993). Alternative views on defining critical thinking through the nursing process. *Holistic Nursing Practice, 7*(3), 71–76.

Jones, A., & Sheppard, L. (2008). Physiotherapy education: A proposed evidence-based model. *Advances in Physiotherapy, 10*(1), 9–13.

Kalischuk, R. G., & Thorpe, K. (2002). Thinking creatively: From nursing education to practice. *The Journal of Continuing Education in Nursing, 33*(4), 155–163.

Karani, R., Leipzig, R., Callahan, E., & Thomas, D. (2004). An unfolding case with a linked objective structured clinical examination (OSCE): A curriculum in inpatient geriatric medicine. *Journal of American Geriatric Society, 52,* 1191–1198.

Keller, J. M. (1987). Development and use of the ARCS model of motivational design. *Journal of Instructional Development, 10*(3), 2–10.

Kelly, C. (2008). Students' perceptions of effective clinical teaching revisited. *Nurse Education Today, 27*(8), 885–892.

Kessler, L., Gielen, A., Diener-West, M., & Paige, D. (1995). The effect of a woman's significant other on her breastfeeding. *Journal of Human Lactation, 11,* 103–109.

Kish, M. H. Z. (2007). Overview of using vignettes to develop higher order thinking and academic achievement in adult learners in an online environment. *International Journal of Information and Communication Technology Education, 2*(3), 60–74.

Klein, J., & Patterson, B. (2008, September 19). Evidence for teaching: What are faculty doing? Paper presented at the NLN Educational Summit, San Antonio, TX.

Knowles, M. (1984). *Andragogy in action: Applying modern principles of adult education.* San Francisco: Jossey-Bass.

Kolb, D. (1976). *Learning style inventory: Technical manual.* Boston: McBer.

Koriat, A. (2008). Easy comes, easy goes? The link between learning and remembering and its exploitation in metacognition. *Memory & Cognition, 36*(2), 416–429.

Koshinen, L. (2004). A nurse's role in mentoring a foreign student. *Sairaanhoitaja, 77*(11), 18–21.

Kruse, K. (n.d.). *Gagne's Nine Events of Instruction: An Introduction.* Retrieved August 2, 2008, from http://www.e-learningguru.com/articles/art3_3.htm

Levett-Jones, T., & Lathlean, J. (2008). Belongingness: A prerequisite for nursing students' clinical learning. *Nurse Education in Practice, 8*(2), 103–111.

Livingston, J. (1997). *Metacognition: An overview.* Retrieved September 27, 2008, from http://www.gse.buffalo.edu/fas/shuell/CEP564/Metacog.htm

Lottes, N. C. (2008). FIRE UP: Tips for engaging student learning. *Journal of Nursing Education, 47*(7), 331–332.

Loughrey, M. (2008). Just how male are male nurses? *Journal of Clinical Nursing, 17*(10), 1327–1334.

Lowe, P., & Kerr, C. (1998). Learning by reflection: The effect on educational outcomes. *Journal of Advanced Nursing, 27,* 1030–1033.

Luse, P. L. (2002). Teaching ideas: Speedwriting: A strategy for active student engagement. *The Reading Teacher, 56*(1), 20–21.

Mangold, K. (2007). Educating a new generation: Teaching baby boomer faculty about millennial students. *Nurse Educator, 32*(1), 21–23.

Mann, A. S. (2004). Eleven tips for the new college teacher. *Journal of Nursing Education, 43*(9), 389–390.

Manstead, A., Proffitt, C., & Smart, J. (1983). Predicting and understanding mothers' infant feeding intentions and behavioral testing the theory of reasoned action. *Journal of Person, Social and Psychology, 44,* 657–671.

Marton, F., & Saljo, R. (1976). On qualitative differences in learning: I—outcome and process. *British Journal of Educational Psychology, 46*(1), 4–11.

McMahon, T. (2006). Teaching for more effective learning: Seven maxims for practice. *Radiography, 12,* 34–44.

Mete, S., & Sari, H. Y. (2008). Nursing students' expectations from tutors in PBL and effects of tutors' behaviour on nursing students. *Nurse Education Today, 28*(4), 434–442.

Miller, M. A., & Malcolm, N. S. (1990). Critical thinking in the nursing curriculum. *Nursing & Healthcare, 11*(2), 66–73.

Milligan, F. (1995). In defense of andragogy. *Nurse Education Today, 15*(1), 22–27.

Mulligan. R. (2007). Management strategies in the educational setting. In B. Moyer & R. A. Wittmann-Price (Eds.), *Teaching nursing: Foundations of practice excellence.* Philadelphia: F.A. Davis Company.

Myrick, F., & Younge, O. (2002). Preceptor behavior integral to the promotion of student critical thinking. *Journal for Nurses in Staff Development, 18*(3), 127–135.

National League for Nursing. (2005). *Core competencies of nurse educators.* Retrieved November 8, 2008, from http://www.nln.org/profdev/pdf/corecompetencies.pdf

Nelms, T. P., Jones, J. M., & Gray, D. P. (1993). Role modeling: A method for teaching caring in nursing education. *Journal of Nursing Education, 32*(1), 18–23.

Nelson, R. (2006). Men in nursing: Still too few, *American Journal of Nursing, 106*(2), 25–26.

Newton, S. (2008). Faculty role modeling of professional writing: One baccalaureate nursing program's experience. *Journal of Professional Nursing, 24*(2), 80–84.

Nilson, L. B. (2003). *Teaching at its best: A research-based resource for college instructors* (2nd ed.). Bolton, MA: Anker Publishing Co.

Nordon, V. (2005). Using music, touch and visual art in developing students communication—why and how? Evaluation of a communication course in a bachelor program in nursing. *Nordic Journal of Nursing Research & Clinical Studies, 25*(4), 47–50.

Novotny, J., & Giffin, M. T. (2006). *A nuts-and-bolts approach to teaching nursing.* New York: Springer Publishing.

Oermann, M. (2004). Using active learning in lecture: Best of "both worlds." *International Journal of Nursing Education Scholarship, 1,* 1–9.

Pardue, K. T., & Morgan, P. (2008). Millennium considered: A new generation, new approaches, and implications for nursing education. *Nursing Education Perspectives, 29*(2), 72–79.

Parker, M. (2005). *Nursing theories and nursing practice* (2nd ed.). Philadelphia: F.A. Davis Company.

Paul, R., & Elder, L. (2007). Critical thinking: The Nature of Critical and Creative Thought. *Journal of Developmental Education, 32*(2), 34–35.

Penney, W., & Warelow, P. (1999). Understanding the prattle of praxis. *Nursing Inquiry, 6,* 259–268.

Pinch, W. J. (1995). Synthesis: Implementing a complex process. *Nurse Educator, 20*(1), 34–40.

Polhemus, L., Swan, K., Danchak, M., & Assis, A. (2005). A Method for Describing Learner Interaction with Content. *Journal of the Research Center for Educational Technology, 1*(2). Retrieved November 8, 2008, from http://www.rcetj.org/?type=art&id=3523&

Quirk, M. E. (1994). *How to learn and teach in medical school: A learner-centered approach.* New York: Charles C. Thomas Publishers.

Ralph, E. (2000). Oral-questioning skills of novice teachers: . . . any questions? *Journal of Instructional Psychology, 26*(4), 286–296.

Ramsden, P., & Entwistle, N. J. (1981). Effects of academic departments on students' approaches to studying. *British Journal of Educational Psychology, 51,* 368–383.

Rankin, S., & Stallings, K. (2001). *Patient education: Principles and practice.* Philadelphia: Lippincott.

Riley-Doucet, C., & Wilson, S. (1997). A three-step method of self-reflection using reflective journal writing. *Journal of Advanced Nursing, 25,* 964–968.

Ross, G., & Tuovinen, J. (2001). Deep versus surface leaning with multimedia in nursing education: Development and evaluation on wound care. *Computers in Nursing, 5,* 213–223.

Rossignol, M. (2000). Verbal and cognitive activities between and among student and faculty in clinical conferences. *Journal of Nursing Education, 39*(6), 245–250.

Rowles, C. J., & Brigham, C. (2005). Strategies to promote critical thinking and active learning. In D. Billings & J. Halstead (Eds.), *Teaching in nursing: A guide for faculty.* St. Louis, MO: Elsevier.

Royse, M. A., & Newton, S. E. (2007). How gaming is used as an innovative strategy for nursing education. *Nursing Education Perspectives, 28*(5), 263–267.

Saunders, R. (2003). Constructing a lesson plan. *Journal for Nurses in Staff Development, 19*(2), 70–78.

Scheffer, B. K., & Rubenfield, M. G. (2000). A consensus statement on critical thinking in nursing. *Journal of Nursing Education, 39*(8), 352–359.

Schon, D. (1983). *The reflective practitioner: How professionals think in action.* New York: Basic Books.

Schunk, D. H., & Zimmerman, B. J. (Eds.). (1994). *Self-regulation of learning and performance.* Hillsdale, NJ: Elbaum.

Schwartz, G., & Cavener, L. A. (1994). Outcome-based education and curriculum change: Advocacy, practice and critique. *Journal of Curriculum and Supervision, 9*(4), 326–338.

Shor, I. (1992). *Empowering education: Critical teaching for social change.* Chicago: University of Chicago Press.

Speakman, E., DeRaineri, J., & Schaal, M. (2008, Sept. 19). *Building bridges for associate degree and diploma graduate by reconceptualizing BSN education for the RN student: Looking at the margins to define the whole.* Paper presented at the meeting of the National League for Nursing Educational Summit, San Antonio, TX.

Staib, S. (2003). Teaching and measuring critical thinking. *Journal of Nursing Education, 42*(11), 498–508.

Starr, C. (2009). Student extra. Lighten up! The use of humor in nursing practice. *American Journal of Nursing, 109*(2), 72AAA–2BBB.

Swanson, V., & Power, K. (2005). Initiation and continuation of breastfeeding: theory of planned behavior. *Journal of Advanced Nursing, 50*(3), 272–282.

Treschuk, J. (2008, September 18). *The art of facilitating collaborative learning.* Paper presented at the meeting of the National League for Nursing Educational Summit, San Antonio, TX.

Turner, P. (2005). Critical thinking in nursing education and practice as defined in the literature. *Nursing Education Perspectives, 26*(5), 272–277.

Tyler, R. W. (1949). *Basic principles of curriculum and instruction.* Chicago: University of Chicago Press.

Van Manen, M. (1991). The concept of pedagogy. In *The tact of teaching: The meaning of pedagogical thoughtfulness.* New York: State University of New York Press.

Vickers, D. A. (2008). Social justice: a concept for undergraduate nursing curricula? *Southern Online Journal of Nursing Research, 2008, 8*(1). Retrieved May 16, 2009, from http://www.nursingplanet.com/Nursing_Research/free_articles3.htm

Vygotsky, L. S. (1978). *Mind in society: The development of higher mental processes.* Belmont, CA: Wadsworth.

Walker, J., Matin, T., White, J., Elliot, R., Norwood, A., & Magnum, C. (2008). Generational (age) differences in nursing student's preferences for teaching methods. *Journal of Nursing Education, 45*(9), 371–374.

Walker, S. (2003). Active learning strategies to promote critical thinking. *Journal of Athletic Training, 38*(3), 263–267.

Watson, G., & Glaser, E. M. (1964). *Critical thinking appraisal.* Orlando, FL: Harcourt, Brace & Jovanovich.

Wetherbee, E., Nordrum, J. T., & Giles, S. (2008). Effective teaching behaviors of APTA-credentialed versus noncredentialed clinical instructors. *Journal of Physical Therapy Education, 22*(1), 65–74.

Weyenberg, D. (1998). The construction of feminist pedagogy in nursing education: A preliminary critique. *Journal of Nursing Education, 37*(8), 345–353.

Wilkenson, J., & Mission, S. (2008, September 18). *Critical thinking: Activities and environment.* Paper presented at the meeting of the National League for Nursing Educational Summit, San Antonio, TX.

Wink, D. (1993). Using questioning as a teaching strategy. *Nurse Educator, 18*(5), 11–15.

Wittmann-Price, R. A. (2007). Promoting reflection in groups of diverse nursing students. In B. Moyer & R. A. Wittmann-Price (Eds.), *Teaching nursing: Foundations of practice excellence*. Philadelphia: F.A. Davis Company.

Wolfe, B. (2007). Men in nursing: Still a frontier, 12–13. Retrieved November 14, 2008, from www.ohnurses.org

Yonge, O., Lee, H., & Luhanga, F. (2006). Closing and not just ending a course. *Nurse Educator, 31*(4), 151–153.

Zsohar, H., & Smith, J. A. (2006). Faculty issues. Top ten list of don'ts in classroom teaching. *Nurse Educator, 31*(4), 144–146.

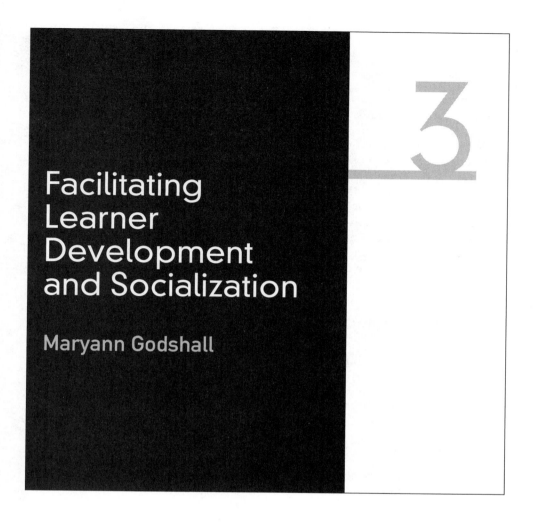

# 3

# Facilitating Learner Development and Socialization

## Maryann Godshall

*Nine tenths of education is encouragement.*

—Anatole France

### NLN Core Competency II: Facilitate Learner Development and Socialization

Nurse educators recognize their responsibility for helping students develop as nurses and integrate the values and behaviors expected of those who fulfill that role (National League for Nursing [NLN], 2005, p. 17).

### Learning Outcomes

- Articulate individual learning styles
- Explore the characteristics of the adult learner
- Investigate Web-based learning
- Examine academic dishonesty and incivility
- Identify ways to incorporate service learning into the curriculum
- Recognize culturally diverse learners
- Identify those with learning disabilities
- Discuss socialization into nursing

## Introduction

Students today present educators with a wide variety of challenges in meeting their educational needs. An educator must take into account a student's cultural, social, and economic background, as well as his or her individual learning style and cognitive ability. These challenges are increased by the need of faculty to assimilate diverse learning environments into teaching, including simulation experiences, online learning, and the integration of new technology into the classroom, including individual student response systems (clickers), blogs, and wiki pages. Added to this is the ever-present need to present information while making the learning environment interactive. This challenges even the most experienced educator. Integrating all of these elements while also incorporating basic education principles is important so that students not only learn, but are also able to pass the NCLEX-RN certification exam when they graduate.

## Assessing Readiness to Learn

Before learning can occur, one must determine if learners are ready to receive the information to be learned (see Table 3.1).

- Readiness to learn occurs when the learner is receptive, willing, and able to participate in the learning process (Bastable, 2008).
- There are five major components to physical readiness; each of these affects learning.
- The components include:
  - Measure of ability
  - Complexity of the task
  - Environmental effects
  - Learner's health status
  - Gender

## Individual Learning Styles

A learning style refers to the ways in which, and conditions under which, learners most efficiently perceive, process, store, and recall what they are attempting to learn (James & Gardner, 1995).

- Cassidy (2004) adds that the approach learners take to different tasks is also important.
- Simply put, a learning style is an approach to learning that works for the individual student.
- Learners may have more than one learning style.
- Educators must first assist learners in identifying their learning style(s), if they do not already know it, and then present information in a manner consistent with the students' learning styles. The four most common learning styles are defined by the acronym VARK, as described by Fleming and Mills (1992).

| Table 3.1 | Four Types of Readiness to Learn | |
|---|---|
| **Type of Readiness** | **Attributes to Assess to Determine Readiness** |
| *P = Physical Readiness* | ■ Measure of ability<br>■ Complexity of the task<br>■ Environmental effects<br>■ Health status<br>■ Gender |
| *E = Emotional Readiness* | ■ Anxiety level<br>■ Support system<br>■ Motivation<br>■ Risk-taking behavior<br>■ Developmental age |
| *E = Experiential Readiness* | ■ Level of aspiration<br>■ Past coping mechanisms<br>■ Cultural background<br>■ Locus of control<br>■ Orientation |
| *K = Knowledge Readiness* | ■ Present knowledge base<br>■ Cognitive ability<br>■ Learning disabilities<br>■ Learning styles |

From *A Self-Study Module of Readiness to Learn,* by C. Lichtenthal, 1990. Unpublished manuscript.

- ■ V = Visual
- ■ A = Auditory
- ■ R = Read/Write
- ■ K = Kinesthetic

## Visual (Spatial) Learners (V)

This type of learner learns best through what they see.

- ■ They like pictures, diagrams, flow charts, time lines, maps, and demonstrations.
- ■ A good learning assignment for a visual learner might involve concept mapping.
- ■ Visual learners like using computers and graphics. These learners could also be called Graphic (G) learners, as this term also explains how they learn.
- ■ It is important to note that visual learners do not learn by viewing movies, videos, or PowerPoint presentations (Fleming, 2001).

# Evidence-Based Education

The Visual Thinking Strategy (VTS) is used to think out loud about an artistic piece of material. Reilly, Ring, and Drake (2005) incorporated this strategy into health-care education and qualitatively found that it increased students' observational skills as well as increased their levels of empathy and sensitivity.

## Aural or Auditory Learners (A)

Aural, or auditory, learners prefer to learn through what is *heard or spoken.*

- These students learn best from lectures, tapes, tutorials, group discussions, speaking, Web chats, e-mail, mobile phones, and talking things through out loud.
- By talking about a topic, these students are able to process the given information (Fleming, 2001).

## Learning by Reading or Writing (R)

These learners prefer to have the information to be learned displayed as *words.*

- These learners prefer text-based input and output in all of its forms.
- Many academics have a preference for this style of learning.
- People with this learning style are often fond of PowerPoint presentations, the Internet, lists, dictionaries, thesauri, quotations, or anything else featuring words (Fleming, 2001).

## Kinesthetic or Active Learners (K)

Kinesthetic, or active, learners use their bodies and sense of touch to enhance learning while engaged in physical activity.

- They like to think about issues while working out or exercising.
- They like to participate, play games, role-play, act, and model experiences through practicing.
- Learning activities tailored to this style could include simulations or real-life experiences.
- Kinesthetic learners appreciate demonstrations, simulations, videos, and movies of "real things," as well as case studies, practice sessions and applications (Fleming, 2001).
- Felder and Solomon (1998) refer to these learners as active learners.

## Multimodal/Mixtures (M)

Multimodal learners are individuals who prefer to learn via two or more styles of learning or using a variety of modes

- These individuals may be context specific or might choose a single mode to suit a certain occasion or situation.
- These individuals like to gather information from each mode and often have a deeper and broader understanding of the topic (Fleming, 2001).

# Other Learning Styles

In addition to the above, there are other learning styles that include:

- Verbal (linguistic) learners
- Tactile learners
- Global learners
- Intuitive learners
- Sequential learners
- Reflective learners
- Analytical learners
- Accommodative learners

## Verbal (Linguistic) Learners

This learning style is an outgrowth of the auditory mode.

- Verbal learners get more value from words that are written or spoken.
- These learners enjoy talking through procedures using a simulator or in clinical practice.
- Verbal learners use recordings of content for repetition.
- These learners frequently write things down or use mnemonics to retain information.

## Tactile Learners

Tactile learners remember what they touch and learn by touching or manipulating objects.

- These learners require movement.
- Tactile learners trace words and use letter tiles to help them learn to spell words.
- Tactile learners love Scrabble.
- Tactile learners often doodle, sketch, write, or conduct experiments (Mahoney, 2007).

## Global Learners

Global learners make decisions based on their emotions and intuition.

- They are spontaneous and focus on creativity.
- A tidy environment is not important to global learners.
- These students enjoy learning. They use humor, tell stories, and enjoy group work.
- Global learners like to participate in activities.
- These learners tend to absorb material randomly. They frequently do not see connections at first, but then suddenly "get it."
- Global learners are able to solve complex problems quickly or put things together in unique ways once they have grasped the big picture, but they may have difficulty explaining how they did it.
- These learners lack good sequential thinking abilities (Felder & Solomon, 1998; Mahoney, 2007).

## Intuitive Learners

These learners like to discover the possibilities in relationships.

- Intuitive learners like solving problems using well-established methods and do not like complications or surprises.
- Intuitive learners do not like repetition.
- These learners tend to work faster and be more innovative than other students.
- Intuitive learners hate courses that involve a lot of memorization or routine calculations and will easily become bored by them.
- Intuitive learners are prone to careless mistakes on tests because they are impatient with details and do not like repetition, such as checking math calculations (Felder & Solomon, 1998).

## Sequential Learners

These learners prefer to gain understanding using linear steps.

- For sequential learners, steps follow one another logically and directly, in an assigned order.
- These learners focus on following a logical sequence to finding solutions (Mahoney, 2007).
- Sequential learners do not like educators who jump from topic to topic or who skip steps.
- Sequential learners like outlines and prefer to follow a defined format (Felder & Solomon, 1998).

## Reflective Learners

A reflective learner prefers to think about new material by reflecting quietly on it first.

- Reflective learners prefer to work alone, rather than with groups.
- These learners do not like classes that cover large amounts of material quickly.
- Reflective learners do not like to be asked simply to read and memorize material.
- These learners like to stop periodically to review what they have read and think of possible questions or applications.
- Reflective learners may find it helpful to write short summaries of readings or class notes in their own words to help them retain the material better (Felder & Solomon, 1998).

## Analytical Learners

These learners base all of their decisions on logic.

- They plan and organize well. They focus on details and facts.
- They like a tidy, well organized environment.
- They enjoy learning, take sequential steps, and follow "the rules."
- They like examples and clear goals (Mahoney, 2007).

## Accommodative Learners

Accommodative learners like a combination of concrete experiences and active experimentation.

- They complete tasks and are less concerned about the theories supporting their actions.
- They are risk takers.
- They solve problems by trial and error.
- They are concerned with abstract concepts and assimilate abstract conceptualizations with reflective observations (Mahoney, 2007).

## Adult Learners

Adult learners display a variety of learning characteristics.

- Malcolm Knowles was one of the first to theorize how adults learn.
- The most common reason an adult enters any learning experience is to create change. This could encompass change in:
  - Their skills
  - Behavior

- Knowledge level
- Their attitudes about things (Russell, 2006)

Barriers to adult learning include:

- Lack of time
- Lack of confidence
- Lack of information about opportunities to learn
- Scheduling problems
- Lack of motivation
- Red-tape (Russell, 2006)

It is important to incorporate adult learning principles into teaching to maximize learning potential for this population. Adult learners learn best when learning is:

- Related to an immediate need, problem, or deficit
- Voluntary and self-initiated
- Person-centered and problem-centered
- Self-controlled and self-directed
- The role of the teacher is that of a facilitator
- Information and assignments are pertinent
- New material draws on past experiences and are related to something the learner already knows
- The learner's perception of threats to him or herself is reduced to a minimum in the educational situation
- Learners are able to participate actively in the learning process
- Students are able to learn in a group
- The nature of the learning activity changes frequently
- Learning is reinforced by application and prompt feedback

## Web-Based Learning

With a decrease of available faculty, the rapid pace of life, and advances in technology, Web-based or online learning is growing in popularity.

- Students like the ability to log on at their convenience.
- Many of the younger, millennial generation's students are hard-wired, always connected to the Internet and are very adept at multi-tasking.
- Many in this generation of learners prefer graphics to text, and prefer Google to the library.
- Contemporary faculty need to integrate these technologies into the classroom and develop an appreciation for and acceptance of this new way of learning.
- Courses may be completely online, or a combination of online and in-class learning. This type of class is referred to as a *hybrid course*.

# Evidence-Based Education

Cook, Gelula, Dupras, and Schwartz (2007) reported that, in a randomized, controlled trial of 89 students that examined Web-based learning and cognitive learning styles (CLS), CLS had no apparent influence on learning outcomes.

The student's role in Web-based learning requires him or her to:

- Be self-directed and self-motivated.
- Be a good written communicator.
- Have access to a reliable computer with reliable Internet access.
- Have the ability to troubleshoot technological issues or computer problems.
- Be able to communicate freely with the instructor and seek help if a problem arises.

The educator's role in a Web-based learning environment requires him or her to:

- Avoid being anxious.
- Develop technological skills.
- Attend technology workshops and seminars.
- Have technological support available (for the educator and students).
- Provide active learning activities.
- Plan in advance.
- Be a facilitator of learning.
- Provide for timely, rich, and prompt feedback.
- Allow for adequate student-faculty interaction time.
- Consider online office hours that are useful to students (offer both virtual and live online office hours).
- Determine and make appropriate assignments:

  - Formative: case studies, critical thinking vignettes, self-tests
  - Summative: written work, games, debates, discussion, portfolios, electronic poster presentations, and tests

- Determine how the course will be evaluated (online evaluation tool).
- Keep an accurate online grade book. This allows students to track their own progress.
- Consider how communication will be managed with students (i.e., via e-mail, discussion boards, and the posting and grading of assignments).
- Establish time-management strategies that include determining the amount of time each day that is to be devoted to each course and responding to student comments.
- Determine how to maintain integrity and deter cheating on tests given online.

(Please see Chapter 6 for more information on Web-based learning.)

## Addressing Incivility

Incivility is defined as "speech or action that is discourteous, rude, or impolite" (Merriam-Webster Online Dictionary, 2008).

- Incivility in the academic nursing environment may range from insulting remarks, verbal abuse, and talking when others are talking to explosive and violent behaviors (Tiberius & Flak, 1999).
- In a study by Luparell (2003), extensive interviews were conducted with 21 nursing professors representing nine nursing programs in six states.
- These faculty all reported that they had been verbally abused by students and that the negative encounters of these experiences were significant and sustained.
- Some faculty questioned their own teaching abilities.
- This topic is so important that it was presented at The National League for Nursing (NLN) Education Summit in 2005, where a lively discussion took place.

A recent study by Clark and Springer (2007) outlines the student behaviors most often reported as incivil by both students and faculty. They are:

- Cheating on examinations or quizzes
- Using cell phones or pagers during class
- Holding distracting conversations
- Making sarcastic remarks or gestures
- Sleeping in class
- Using computers for purposes not related to the class
- Demanding make-up examinations, extensions, or other favors
- Making disapproving groans
- Dominating class discussions
- Refusing to answer direct questions

Incivility is a symptom of a larger problem of academic dishonesty, which is defined as the "intentional participation in deceptive practices regarding one's academic work or the work of another" (Kolanko et al., 2006, p. 1).

- As many as 70% to 95% of students reported having engaged in practices of academic dishonesty.
- Some have suggested that the problem of academic dishonesty is a result of a deterioration in morals, as reported over the past decade by the Joseph Institute (Kolanko et al., 2006).

Students described the following behaviors as *ineffective* for deterring cheating:

- Assigning specific topics for papers
- Putting numbers on test booklets

- Assigning seats for exams
- Permitting only pencils to be brought into the exam room
- Not permitting anyone to leave during the course of the exam
- Leaving increased space between students during an exam

Students describe the following behaviors as *most* effective in deterring cheating:

- Having students place their belongings in the front of the classroom
- Having a minimum of two proctors per exam to walk up and down the aisles during the exam
- Providing new exams for each test
- Keeping each test in a locked cabinet with shredding conducted by full-time secretaries, not student aids.

Kolanko et al. (2006) also noted that "faculty should include opportunities within the education process for the moral development of students in addition to their theoretical and clinical development.

- Students must understand what constitutes academic integrity.
- Unethical behavior is ultimately responsible for the deterioration of the very fabric of the nursing profession" (p. 35).

It is also important to note that incivility can flow from the faculty member to the student. Faculty must always be aware of their behavior and their position as role models for students. Unfortunately, Clark (2006) found that it is not unusual for students to perceive faculty as uncivil. Her study found uncivil faculty behaviors to include:

- Making demeaning and belittling comments
- Treating students unfairly
- Pressuring students to conform to unreasonable faculty demands.

Faculty members arriving unprepared and late for class can also be considered uncivil, and any of the characteristics identified as uncivil student behaviors may also be applied to faculty. Three themes emerged from Clark's study related to students' emotional responses to faculty incivility. They included feeling:

- Traumatized,
- Powerless and helpless, and
- Angry

As these studies reveal, uncivil behavior is a double-edged sword and must be examined and remedied at both ends of the learning continuum.

## Service Learning

Nursing is an interactive and caring discipline. Implementation of service learning is a way for students to give back to the community through a partnership that delivers a needed service (Wittmann-Price, 2008). Vaderhoff (2005) defines service learning as "giving students the opportunity to provide service to others while tying in learning objectives and a class project for professional development" (p. 36).

- It is important to realize that service learning is more than simple community service. It is a course-based educational experience for credit (Bentley & Ellison, 2005).
- Service learning can be done locally or internationally.
- The setting for service learning may vary.
- It can be used to enhance cultural competence for students in a variety of settings (Wittmann-Price, 2008). (For more information about service learning, please see Chapter 7.)

## Culturally Diverse Students

The culture of the individual encompasses an individual's values, attitudes, perceptions, interpersonal needs, roles, and cognitive styles (Tomey, 2009). It is important for faculty to recognize that cultural diversity can influence learning ability and needs when teaching nursing students and when socializing them into the role of a nurse. Additionally, diversity may influence how nursing is perceived by individuals from diverse alternative cultural backgrounds. For example, a nurse who, in one culture, may be considered a "caring nurse" may be perceived by members of another culture as cold and aloof. Perceptions of individuals must be considered from each individual's cultural background.

The American Association of Colleges of Nursing (AACN) issued a position statement in 1997 stating that, because the United States' population is so culturally diverse, cultural diversity training needs to be included in nursing education and a greater number of culturally diverse students should be recruited into nursing schools (American Association of Colleges of Nursing, 1997). Despite this position statement, minorities continue to be under-represented in nursing and nursing programs (Wellman, 2009). Moreover, culturally diverse students face certain barriers that may impinge on their ability to achieve success in college. The most common of these barriers are:

- The lack of ethnically diverse faculty
- Finances
- Academic preparation (Wellman, 2009)

Culturally diverse students may also suffer from a lack of:

- Available role models
- Academic support
- Family support
- Peer support

## Culturally Diverse Learners

The culture or customs of an individual nursing student or individual learner may, at times, come into conflict with the values of the clinical environment and his or her values system may be disrupted.

- A value represents a basic conviction about what is right, wrong, desirable, or just, and may support an individual's decision about how to act or perform in relation to what is perceived as preferable or valuable within the individual's culture.
- This can contribute to forming attitudes, which are similar to values that are learned from the individual's parents, caregivers, and family.
- Teachers and peers may have a significant impact on one's actions.
- Some students may experience a situation that differs from the values of their cultural tradition and usual behavior, thus causing them to experience cognitive dissonance.
- The inconsistencies revealed by cognitive dissonance are both uncomfortable and ambiguous for students (Tomey, 2009).
- It is important, especially for nursing educators, to offer clear directions and rationale for decision making for culturally diverse students to help alleviate any sense of dissonance they might experience.

A study by Amaro et al. (2006) interviewed ethnically diverse students who had recently completed an Associate or Baccalaureate nursing program and identified the major themes related to educational barriers. These include:

- Personal needs (lack of finances, time issues, family responsibilities and obligations, and difficulties related to language and communication)
- Academic needs (large or heavy workload)
- Language needs (difficulty reading and understanding assignments, a prejudice due to their accents, verbal communication barriers)
- Cultural needs (expectations related to assertiveness and cultural norms, lack of diverse role models, and difficulty with communication)

An important issue among culturally diverse learners is their level of knowledge of the English language, which, if inadequate, can be problematic. Barriers may also exist for the English as a Second Language (ESL) student in applying and gaining admission to nursing programs and in their ability to progress through the program, once accepted.

Suggestions for accommodating students from culturally and linguistically diverse backgrounds include:

- Using non-standardized and standardized methods of testing
- Dynamic assessments
- Nonverbal measures of ability
- Multiple methods of testing
- Testing in both the learner's native and second language
- The use of the TOEFL® test (Overton, Felding, & Simonsson, 2004)

## The TOEFL® Examination

The Test of English as a Foreign Language (TOEFL®) examination measures a learner's potential ability to communicate in English in a college or university environment.

- The TOEFL score can be helpful in identifying students who may be at risk for failure and/or may need additional support throughout a program (Educational Testing Services, 2008).
- It is important to use the TOEFL score as only one piece of admission criteria.
- Be aware that students may be offended if they are asked to take a TOEFL exam if they have been living in the United States for many years.

Faculty commitment to the success of minority students is crucial for the success of diverse student populations. Minority students need a strong student-faculty relationship with a faculty member who is not responsible for assigning a grade to the student.

Stolder, Rosemeyer, and Zorn (2008) tell about a respite care for students program that is a partnership program with a community healthcare agency. The program is designed to assist students who have low social support and to encourage them to Take a Break (TAB). This program has increased retention of students and is especially beneficial to students who have demanding external responsibilities.

- Students need someone to talk to about their feelings and experiences as they move through the nursing program.
- Having strong student-faculty relationships will minimize students' experiences with cognitive dissonance.
- Role models are ideal if appropriate faculty candidates are available.
- If no faculty role model is found, other faculty members must spend time with these students to ensure their success (Wellman, 2009).

Developing adequate support services for culturally diverse students will increase their success in nursing or other academic programs. Reading, comprehension, and writing skills need to be developed in a non-threatening manner to assist the diverse student's academic success. (For further information on culturally diverse students, please see Chapter 4.)

## Learning Disabilities

Learning disabilities are the most common type of student disability found on college campuses. Frequently students with a learning disability begin college without their disability having been detected.

- In nursing education, these disabilities are often noted when significant differences are noticed between a student's classroom and clinical performance.
- Often, a student may perform well in the clinical area, but may be unable to demonstrate the same ability, skills, and competency when taking tests in the classroom.
- These students should be referred to the appropriate counselors for assistance (Frank, 2009).

Learners with documented disabilities are entitled to the same access to education as traditional students. An office of academic services must be available to provide learners with reading, writing, and test-taking strategy support services.

## The Elementary and Secondary Education Act

The Elementary and Secondary Education Act was passed in 1965 to "ensure equal educational opportunity for all children . . . and to close the achievement gap between poor and affluent children" (No Child Left Behind Act [NCLB], 2001, Sec. 1001). This has since undergone changes and has most recently been enhanced by the No Child Left Behind Act of 2001.

## The No Child Left Behind Act (NCLB)

The No Child Left Behind Act (NCLB) is the most significant federal education policy in a generation. The Act calls on all educators to measure all students' performances using a set of fixed indicators and has tied federal monetary compensation to these performance outcomes.

It should be noted that, while these laws are aimed at elementary and secondary education, it cannot be ignored and will have tremendous impact when these students taught under the auspices of the acts reach college. Educators should be prepared for challenges yet to be determined that may stem from these acts, especially NCLB (Nagel, Yunker, & Malmgren, 2006).

Some of the characteristics of students with learning disabilities are:

- Trouble with basic reading skills
- Memory difficulties
- Trouble remembering details and sequencing
- Reading and spelling difficulties
- Poor handwriting
- Distractibility with difficulty concentrating
- History of poor academic performance
- Difficulty meeting deadlines
- Anxiety and low self-esteem
- Difficulty following verbal instructions
- Difficulty organizing ideas into writing
- Inability to articulate ideas verbally, but can articulate them in writing
- Auditory processing deficits
- Time management problems (Frank, 2009)

It is important for faculty to know that the nature of learning disabilities can be highly individualized and can be manifest differently through the grouping of a variety of issues. Some characteristics shared by these students can include any of the following:

- These students are usually of average or above average intelligence (Frank, 2009).

- Employing teaching strategies that match the student's learning style may enhance students' chance of success and may serve to minimize their learning disability.
- The skilled educator is aware and open to employing teaching strategies to assist learning disabled students to achieve.

Many colleges and universities have an office that coordinates the diagnosis of learning disabilities and the accommodation and provision of support services for students who need them.

- If a student agrees, a faculty member can be made aware of the student's disability and a variety of accommodations can be made to meet the student's learning needs. One example involves giving the student extra time to take an exam or allowing the student to take an exam in another secured environment.
- It is not appropriate for the faculty to discuss a student's learning disability with other faculty members unless given permission to do so by the student (Frank, 2009).

Nurse educators must also be familiar with the accommodations made by their state for students with disabilities. The National Council Licensure Examination (NCLEX-RN) has accommodations for students with documented learning disabilities.

- Accommodations must be made for students with learning disabilities in accordance with the Americans with Disabilities Act (National Council of States Boards of Nursing, 2009).
- It is important for educators to be aware of students with physical disabilities, such as students with a documented or apparent physical limitation, substance abuse, chemical or alcohol impairments, and/or mental health problems (Frank, 2009).

## Student Socialization

Socialization is defined as a process of internalizing the norms, beliefs, and values of a professional culture to which one hopes to gain admission (Philipin, 1999).

- New nurses are instructed in ways and attitudes of the organization and gradually adopt the attitudes, values, and unspoken messages within the organization (Mooney, 2007).
- It is important to note that a lack of socialization to nursing has been associated with negative outcomes such as turnover, attrition from the profession, and decreased productivity (Nesler, Hanner, Melbur, & McGowen, 2001).

Kramer's work delineates four phases of what is described as "reality shock" when a new nurse or neophyte realizes what he or she learned in school does not match that which is experienced in actual clinical practice.

- The excitement of passing the licensure examination quickly passes as these new nurses struggle to move from the role of student to the staff nurse role.
- This reality shock leads to stress, which can cause exacerbations of symptoms that affect one's health and cause a loss of time from work (Cherry & Jacob, 2005).

Kramer's Four Phases of Reality Shock include:

1. Honeymoon
2. Shock or rejection
3. Recovery
4. Resolution

## Benner's Novice to Expert Theory

Patricia Benner (1984) discussed this same issue in her "from novice to expert nurses" theory. The phases she outlined are:

1. Novice
2. Advanced Beginner
3. Competent
4. Proficient
5. Expert

It is important to note that socialization takes place primarily through social interaction with people who are significant to an individual, usually a nursing school's faculty members (Barretti, 2004). In the hospital environment, the following contributed to the successful socialization of new nursing graduates as they developed self-confidence and high role-satisfaction (Boyle, Popkess-Vawter, & Taunton, 1996):

- Positive precepting experiences
- Social support systems
- Assignment congruence

What nurse educators can do to enhance student socialization into nursing is two-fold.

- First, a nurse educator should be a great role model for the profession.
- Second, a nurse educator should prepare nursing students for the reality of the profession by integrating socialization principles into every nursing course in the curriculum.

Nursing educators today are shaping tomorrow's nurses. What is paramount to the successful shaping of tomorrow's nursing staff is that nurse educators not only teach nursing content, but also shape the learning environment where that content is taught, including appropriate clinical experiences, so that students are fully socialized to the reality of nursing and its role. Accomplishing this will serve to reduce the chance of negative experiences and reality shock upon graduation.

# Evidence-Based Practice

Within the first year of employment, turnover rate for newly graduated nurses ranges from 30% to 60%. A study of perceptions of the work environment and job satisfaction of new nurses in their first 18 months of employment found that nurses' intent to stay was linked to aspects of scheduling, coworker and physician relationships, professional growth opportunities, recognition, control, and responsibility (Halfer & Graff, 2006).

# CASE STUDIES

## Case Study 3.1

You are the instructor in a 12-month accelerated nursing program. Due to the time constraints of only having the students for 12 months, you realize it is essential to incorporate only the most important facts in your course. Your program has successfully graduated four groups of accelerated students. Your university sends out a follow-up survey to see how these students are doing in the clinical environment. On the surveys you see comments like, "I didn't realize nursing was going to be this hard; I wasn't really ready for the demands of working in this fast-paced environment; I didn't think it would be this hard fitting in on the floor where I work; No one really helps me; I am not sure I am going to remain in nursing; I wish I knew it was going to be like this." You realize that, perhaps by focusing so much on getting in all the content needed for students to pass their licensure exams, your university missed out on providing an important lesson. Your program did not take the time to "socialize" these students to the role of nursing. List some ideas of how you might better address the socialization of nursing students in the future, in both your course and at the university level.

## Case Study 3.2

You have been teaching for the past three years in a university setting. Your class typically has 50 students and meets in a large auditorium. You try to keep the students engaged and actively involved in the learning process, but frequently you notice that students are talking amongst themselves while you are teaching. Is this an example of students being uncivil? If so, what might you do to curtail this in the classroom?

# Case Study 3.3

You are teaching a course that has a clinical component. You notice that a particular student does exceptionally well in the clinical area. She is professional, completes excellent assessments, and interacts beautifully with the patients. In the classroom, however, this student seems to be the last one done when taking a test, and is barely passing the course. What do you think is going on with this student? What would you do to help her? Do you think this student may have a learning disability? Answer yes or no, and support your answer.

# Practice Questions

1. A nurse educator is designing a program to assist culturally diverse learners in your university's courses. Which of the following strategies would be most beneficial for the educator to include?
   A. Obtaining monetary assistance for student scholarships
   B. Offering a one-on-one orientation session for each course
   C. Holding study group sessions limited to culturally diverse learners
   D. Developing a mentor program that pairs learners with a faculty member.

2. A nurse educator is teaching an online course about the concepts of nursing. One of the learners has posted an opinion to the discussion board that is negative about the profession of nursing. Other students in the class have posted comments in agreement with the first posting. What should the nurse educator teaching the course do?
   A. Do nothing and let the situation blow over.
   B. Courteously question the student's first posting and open a dialogue about the topic.
   C. Post evidence-based research to prove the student wrong.
   D. Remind the student that negative posts will be deleted.

3. A nurse educator recognizes that a student who is a visual learner would prefer which of the following assignments:
   A. Watch a movie and then discuss it with the class.
   B. Read a textbook and write an essay
   C. Create a concept map using a computer
   D. Perform the skill in a simulation lab

4. The best example of a service learning project would be
   A. Collecting blankets for the homeless
   B. Participating in a teddy bear clinic for course credit
   C. Helping to decorate for local foster children's Christmas party
   D. Attending a meeting to plan community outreach programs

5. A student does poorly on an exam and then approaches the educator to share that they have attention deficit hyperactivity disorder (ADHD). The student asks the educator if, in the future, they may take tests in another room and be given more time. What would be the best response to the student by the educator?
   A. "Why did you not come to me about this before you took the test?"
   B. "Do you have a note from the learning center verifying this disorder?"

    C.  Ask the student if they feel this disorder is affecting their performance in the classroom and during testing.

    D.  "You may come to my office to take the test, using as much time as you need."

6.  A student has made a medication error in the clinical area during the pediatric rotation. The nurse educator could best demonstrate "role modeling" of the nursing profession and good socialization skills by doing which of the following?

    A.  Make the student go to the primary nurse and director to tell them she made a mistake.

    B.  Take the student aside in a private area to review the error made, notify the appropriate individuals, and fill out an internal incident report.

    C.  Tell the entire group about the mistake in a post-conference session. Use it as a learning experience for all as to what not to do.

    D.  Send the student home from the clinic and then draft a learning contract.

7.  Which of the following is an example of an uncivil behavior by a student in the classroom? (Choose all that apply.)

    A.  Talking to another student while the instructor is lecturing

    B.  Asking the educator for permission to leave the classroom during an exam because they feel ill

    C.  Wearing a baseball hat to class during an exam

    D.  Asking a question of a teacher and then arguing with him or her, saying that the response is inaccurate

8.  Which of the following phases is described by a student who just passed her licensure examination, is off of orientation, and is in her third week of taking a solo patient assignment in the critical care unit? Suddenly, her patient deteriorates so she asks a senior nurse for help. The senior nurse responds, "Why don't you go ask your preceptor, I am too busy."

    A.  Honeymoon

    B.  Shock or rejection

    C.  Recovery

    D.  Resolution

9.  A novice educator just attended a conference on utilizing technology in an online course. Soon, she will be teaching her first online course. Which of the following statements would indicate the novice educator's need for additional learning?

    A.  "I am so confident, I am going to use all of these technologies learned and I won't need any more technological help, what a relief!"

    B.  "My main priority is to keep a good line of communication open with my students."

    C.  "I need to make sure my online students can access the databases from home as easily as the on-campus students can."

    D.  "I would like to integrate YouTube video clips into the learning environment."

10. In understanding cultural diversity of students in the classroom. You wrote a test question in which the best answer was for the student to choose a clear liquid to give the patient. During the exam, a Chinese student with English as a second language approaches you to ask you what "Gatorade" is. An astute educator should do which of the following:
    A. Be aware the student is being uncivil and trying to get the answer.
    B. Realize that "Gatorade" is not a good example of a clear liquid.
    C. Realize that not all cultures are familiar with American food and drink, such as Gatorade as a clear liquid.
    D. Tell the student to sit down and choose the best answer.

# References

Amaro, D. J., Abriam-Yago, K., & Yoder, M. (2006). Perceived barriers for ethnically diverse students in nursing programs. *Journal of Nursing Education, 45*(7), 247–254.

American Association of Colleges of Nursing. (1997). *Diversity and equality of opportunity.* Washington, DC Author.

Barretti, M. (2004). What do we know about the professional socialization of our students? *Journal of Social Work Education, 40*(2), 255–283.

Bastable, S. B. (2008). *Nurse as educator: Principles of teaching and learning from nursing practice* (3rd ed.). Boston: Jones and Bartlett Publishers.

Benner, P. (1984). *From novice to expert: Excellence and power in clinical nursing practice.* Boston: Addison-Wesley.

Bentley, R., & Ellison, K. (2005). Impact of service-learning projects on nursing students. *Nursing Education Perspectives, 26*(5), 287–290.

Boyle, D. K., Popkess-Vawter, S., & Taunton, R. L. (1996). Socialization of new graduate nurses in critical care. *Heart & Lung, 25* (2), 141–154.

Cassidy, S. (2004). Learning styles: An overview of theories, models, and measures. *Educational Psychology, 24*(4), 419–444.

Cherry, B., & Jacob, S. R. (2005). *Contemporary nursing: Issues, trends, and management.* St. Louis, MO: Elsevier.

Clark, C. M. (2006). *Incivility in nursing education: student perceptions of uncivil faculty behavior in the academic environment.* Unpublished Doctoral dissertation, University of Idaho.

Clark, C. M., & Springer, P. J. (2007). Incivility in nursing education: A descriptive study of definitions and prevalence. *Journal of Nursing Education, 46*(1), 7–14.

Cook, D. A., Gelula, M. H., Dupras, D. M., & Schwartz, A. (2007). Instructional methods and learning styles in web-based learning: Report of two randomized trials. *Medical Education, 41,* 897–905.

Educational Testing Services. (2008). *The TOEFL® Test.* Retrieved December 1, 2008, from http://www.toeflgoanywhere.org/

Felder, R. M., & Solomon, B. A. (1998). Learning styles and strategies. Retrieved November 28, 2008, from http://www4.ncsu.edu/unity/lockers/users/f/felder/public/ILSdir/styles.htm

Fleming, N. (2001). VARK: A guide to learning styles. Retrieved November 28, 2008, from http://www.vark-learn.com/english/page.asp?p = categories

Fleming, N., & Mills, C. (1992). Not another inventory, rather a catalyst for change. In D. Wulff & J. Nygist (Eds.), *To improve the academy: Resources for faculty, instructional, and organizational development* (Vol. 11, pp. 137–155). Stillwater, OK: New Forums, Inc.

Frank, B. (2009). Teaching students with disabilities. In D. M. Billings & J. A. Halstead (Eds.), *Teaching in nursing: A guide for faculty* (pp. 18–31). St. Louis, MO: Mosby/Elsevier.

Halfer, D., & Graf, E. (2006). Graduate nurse perception of the work experience. *Nursing Economics, 24*(3), 150–155.

James, W. B., & Gardner, D. L. (1995). Learning styles: Implications for distance learning. *New Directions for Adult and Continuing Education, 67*(1), 19–32.

Kolanko, K. M., Clark, C., Heinrich, K. T., Olive, D., Serembus, J. F., & Sifford, K. S. (2006). Academic dishonesty, bullying, incivility, and violence: Difficult challenges facing nurse educators. *Nursing Education Perspectives, 27*(1), 34–43.

Lichtenthal, C. (1990). *A self-study module of readiness to learn.* Unpublished manuscript.

Luparell, S. M. (2003). Critical incidents of incivility by nursing students: How uncivil encounters with students affect nursing faculty (Doctoral dissertation, University of Nebraska, 2003). *Dissertation Abstracts International, 64,* 2128.

Mahoney, P. (2007). *Certified Nurse Educator preparation course.* Philadelphia: Villanova University.

Merriam-Webster Online Dictionary. (2008). *Incivility.* Retrieved December 2, 2008, from http://www.merriam-webster.com/dictionary/incivility

Mooney, M. (2007). Professional socialization: The key to survival as a newly qualified nurse. *International Journal of Nursing Practice, 13,* 75–80.

Nagle, K., Yunker, C., & Malmgren, K. W. (2006). Students with disabilities and accountability reform. *Journal of Disability Policy Studies, 17*(1), 28–39.

National Council of State Boards of Nursing (2009). NCLEX Exam Process Overview. Retrieved May 1, 2009, from http://www.ncsbn.org

National League for Nursing (NLN). (2005). *Core competencies of nurse educators.* Retrieved November 8, 2008, from http://www.nln.org/profdev/pdf/corecompetencies.pdf

Nesler, M. S., Hanner, M. B., Melburg, V., & McGowan, S. (2001). Professional socialization of baccalaureate nursing students: can students in distance nursing programs become socialized? *Journal of Nursing Education, 40*(7), 293–302.

No Child Left Behind Act (NCLB). P. L. 107–110, 115 stat. 1425 (2001).

Overton, T., Fielding, C., & Simonsson, M. (2004). Decision making in determining eligibility of culturally and linguistically diverse learners. *Journal of Learning Disabilities, 37*(4), 319–330.

Philipin, S. M. (1999). The impact of project 2000 educational reforms on the occupational socialization of nurses: An exploratory study. *Journal of Advanced Nursing, 29*(6), 1326–1331.

Reilly, J. M., Ring, J., & Drake, L. (2005). Visual thinking strategies: A new role for art in medical education. *Family Medicine, 37*(4), 250–252.

Russell, S. S. (2006). An overview of adult learning. *Urologic Nursing, 26*(5), 349–370.

Stolder, M. E., Rosemeyer, A. K., & Zorn, C. R. (2008). In the shelter of each other: respite care for students as a partnership model. *Nursing Education Perspectives, 29*(5), 295–299.

Tiberius, R. G., & Flak, E. (1999). Incivility in dyadic teaching and learning. *New Directions for Teaching and Learning, 77,* 3–12.

Tomey, A. M. (2009). *Nursing management and leadership* (8th ed.). St. Louis, MO: Mosby/Elsevier.

Vanderhoff, M. (2005, May). Service learning: The world as a classroom. *PT Magazine,* 34–41.

Wellman, D. S. (2009). The diverse learning needs of students. In D. M. Billings & J. A. Halstead (Eds.), *Teaching in nursing: A guide for faculty* (pp. 18–31). St. Louis, MO: Mosby/Elsevier.

Wittmann-Price, R. A. (2008). Promoting reflection in groups of diverse nursing students. In B. A. Moyer & R. A. Wittmann-Price (Eds.), *Nursing education: Foundations for practice* (pp. 231–243). Philadelphia: F.A. Davis Company.

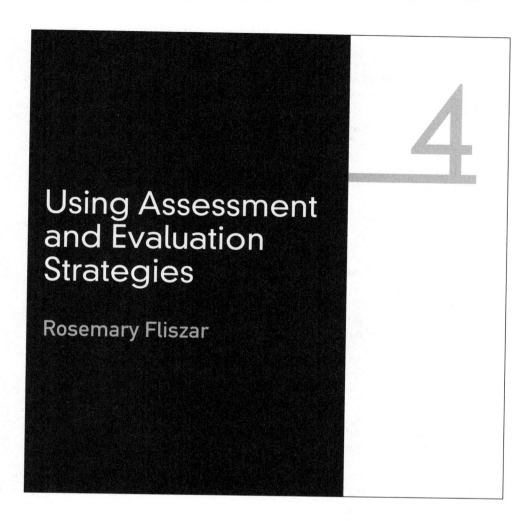

# Using Assessment and Evaluation Strategies

Rosemary Fliszar

*Learning without thought is labor lost.*

—Confucius

**NLN Core Competency III: Use Assessment and Evaluation Strategies**

Nurse educators use a variety of strategies to assess and evaluate student learning in classroom, laboratory and clinical settings, as well as in all domains of learning (National League for Nursing [NLN], 2005, p. 18).

**Learning Outcomes**

Identify internal and external factors influencing admission, progression, and graduation in a nursing program.

- Utilize nursing program standards related to admission and progression.
- Describe the process of program evaluation to assess outcomes in a nursing curriculum.

- Use a variety of strategies to assess learning in the cognitive, affective, and psychomotor domains.
- Understand various frameworks and models upon which evaluation and assessment is based.
- Analyze assessment and evaluation data in determining achievement of learner and program outcomes.
- Use assessment and evaluation data to enhance the teaching-learning process and influence program outcomes.

## Introduction

This chapter will focus on the factors that influence nursing education program outcomes. The relationship of standards related to admission and progression within the parent institution in general, and the nursing program in particular, will be discussed. Methods of assessing learning and outcomes will be presented to provide a mechanism for the nurse educator to determine program effectiveness and identify strategies to improve the quality of the nursing program.

## Definitions

In order to understand the assessment and evaluation process involved in a nursing education program, it is important to understand the terminology related to this process.

- "[A] nursing education program refers to any academic program offered in a postsecondary education institution which results in initial licensure or advanced preparation in nursing" (Sauter, Johnson, & Gillespie, 2009, p. 467).
  - Nursing programs that offer initial licensure are of three types:
    - Baccalaureate degree—A 4-year program offered by a college or university
    - Associate degree—A 2-year program typically offered by a community college
    - Diploma—A 2- or 3-year program that is hospital-based and offered in a School of Nursing
  - Nursing programs offering advanced preparation in nursing occur at the college or university level and include:
    - RN-BSN programs
    - RN-MSN programs
    - MSN degree
    - Doctorate
- Program evaluation refers to "the assessment of all components of the program" (Sauter, Johnson, & Gillespie, 2009, p. 467).

- "Standards are rules for the measurement of quality, extent, value, and quantity" (NLNAC Accreditation Manual, 2008, p. 10).
- "Criteria are statements that define the variables to examine in evaluation of a standard" (NLNAC Accreditation Manual, 2008, p. 10).

## Standards of the University/College/Nursing Program

The *admission* policies of an institution are the first standards with which a student is evaluated for admission into a nursing program. The policies must be clearly defined and published by the institution. The nursing program in an academic setting may further refine these standards and criteria to ensure the academic quality of the students entering the program. Criteria for admission into a nursing program may include:

- Standardized testing, such as the Scholastic Aptitude Test (SAT) for undergraduate education and Graduate Record Examinations (GRE) for graduate applications
- Courses taken in high school or college with a strong science and math base
- Minimum Grade Point Average (GPA)
- Personal letter of intent
- Letters of reference
- Background checks (Farnsworth & Springer, 2006)

Success of students on the National Council of Licensure Examinations—Registered Nurse (NCLEX-RN) examination is the benchmark for all nursing programs for achieving minimum standards of competency and quality. Predictive criteria have been studied to determine the attributes of a nursing student necessary for passing the NCLEX-RN. Yin and Burger (2003) found that the following criteria were excellent predictors of which students enrolled in an Associate Degree nursing program would successfully pass the NCLEX-RN:

- College GPA prior to admission into the nursing program was found to be the most important predictor of success.
- High GPAs in natural science courses—biology, chemistry, and anatomy and physiology
- Course grade in an introductory psychology course
- High school rank

Sayles, Shelton, and Powell (2003) found that other predictors, in addition to the above, also improved success rates of students on the NCLEX-RN:

- Scores on the Nurse Entrance Test (NET) Comprehensive Achievement Profiles administered by Educational Resources, Inc.
- Pre-RN Assessment scores

High GPAs in the natural sciences and other college courses taken prior to admission into baccalaureate nursing programs have also been predictive of student success when taking the NCLEX-RN. Based on this success rate, many nursing programs of all three types now require students to complete all college requirements prior to admission into a nursing program. Admission into the nursing major has become very selective based on specific criteria as identified by the individual nursing program. In a Baccalaureate program with this admission requirement, students enter the nursing major at the junior level if they have met the strict criteria for admission into the program.

Admission criteria for graduate nursing education must be clearly developed for applicants to this program. The policies must be congruent with the institution's policy, but, as is seen in undergraduate education, they may be more selective for admission into the nursing program. Predictors of success in a graduate program have been based on the undergraduate GPA and scores on the Graduate Record Exam (GREs). However, Newton and Moore (2007) found that undergraduate GPA was not always predictive of success when taking GREs and, as such, should be used with caution when making decisions related to admission into a graduate nursing program. Many nursing programs waive the standardized testing requirement if applicants have a GPA of 3.3 or 3.5 or greater.

## Evidence-Based Education

Dela Cruz and Klakovich (2008) have studied career transitions into nursing using Schlossberg's Transition Framework and highlighting the concepts of moving into the learning environment, moving through it, and preparing to leave. Elements of the curriculum that promoted career transition included: providing preadmission counseling, emphasizing professional knowledge, and introducing the student to professional employment. These curriculum changes were successful in increasing the NCLEX-RN pass rates from 96% to 100%.

## Progression Policies

Progression policies within the nursing major must be congruent with the program goals and institutional standards, and must be clearly identified and published. Criteria that are often included in progression policies include:

- Minimum course grades for nursing and science courses
- Minimum cumulative GPA for progression in the program
- Number of times a student may repeat selective courses at both the undergraduate and graduate levels
- Standards in place if a student takes a leave of absence during the program of study
- Achievement of a minimum grade on standardized achievement tests such as HESI or ATIs based on established benchmarks for prelicensure RN students

# The Evaluation/Assessment Process

Evaluation is the process of systematically collecting and analyzing data that has been gathered through various measurements in order to determine the merit, worth, and value of something and to render a judgment about the subject of the evaluation (Mahara, 1998; O'Connor, 2006). Evaluation in the educational setting is conducted to determine (1) student progress toward achieving program outcomes, (2) effectiveness of the educational process to foster student learning, and (3) accomplishment of the mission of the institution to prepare nurses for entry into practice (O'Connor, 2006).

Assessment is the process of obtaining information about students, faculty, programs, and institutions, and is often used interchangeably with the term evaluation. More specifically, assessment involves setting standards and criteria for learning, gathering, analyzing, and interpreting data to determine how performance matches the standards and criteria, and to use that information to improve student learning, teaching, courses, and programs (Angelo, 1993; Bourke & Ihrke, 2009).

> Clinical instructors must make two professional judgments about student performance—whether the student has met course objectives and whether the student can safely provide care (Orchard, 1994).

## Philosophies of Evaluation

The evaluation process is influenced by the evaluator's beliefs about evaluation and their philosophical perspective. Some examples of evaluation philosophies include:

- Practice orientation
  - Practice goals are reflected in course objectives.
  - Performance achieved at the end of the course, clinical experience, or program is the most important consideration.
- Service orientation
  - This perspective is based on a values approach to evaluation.
  - This view takes a more global or holistic view of the goals of the educational process beyond course objectives.
  - This perspective includes goals that are integrated into a model of performance that represents the typical or ideal student at a particular level of development.
  - With this approach, instructors view the evaluation process as a means to identify student strengths and weaknesses in various components of performance. Guides the facilitation of student progress toward model performance.
- Judgment orientation
  - This perspective reflects a focus on the determination of acceptability of student performance and the value or grade that should be assigned based on the performance.
  - Instructors assign a pass/fail grade or letter and numerical grading—pass/fail is used most often in clinical grading.

- Constructivist orientation
  - Assigns heaviest consideration to stakeholders who will be affected by the success or failure of the program. In nursing, the stakeholders are the employers of graduates and the recipients of the graduates' nursing care.
  - The evaluation process involves input from patients and staff who contribute to the assignment of the grade in the clinical setting (O'Connor, 2006).

> The best test combines aspects of both norm-referenced and criterion-referenced tests.

## Purposes of Evaluation

The purpose of the evaluation process must be clearly delineated for faculty and students. Purposes of evaluation include:

- Identification of learning
- Diagnosis of problems, such as learning needs or deficits in teaching practices, courses, or the curriculum
- Decision-making related to assignment of grades, tenure, and promotion
- Improvement of products, such as textbooks or course content
- Judgment of effectiveness of student goal achievement and the meeting of standards and program outcomes (Bourke & Ihrke, 2009; O'Connor, 2006)

## Formative Evaluation

- Refers to the evaluation of learning while it is occurring
- Identifies a student's readiness to learn and learning needs
- May be used to improve student performance before the end of the course or program
- Assigns no final grade
- Shares the evaluation with the student informally throughout the learning process, but formally presented in clinical courses at mid-semester

## Summative Evaluation

- Refers to the level of performance of the student at the end of the course, program, or activity
- Makes judgment as to whether or not the standards and criteria have been met for the event (course, clinical, program)
- Uses data collected throughout the learning experience as the basis for evaluation
- Assigns a final grade (letter, numeric, pass/fail, satisfactory/unsatisfactory)
- Evaluator determines evaluation and shares with the student being evaluated while the summative period is in effect, particularly in clinical courses or activities

## Evaluation Models

An evaluation model is useful for explaining the process upon which variables, items, or events are evaluated, and provides a systematic plan or framework for evaluation. Several models are used in nursing education, and should be selected based on the context, needs of stakeholders, and the question to be evaluated. Some of the evaluation models are included here (Bourke & Ihrke, 2009):

- Logic Model
    - Useful in designing program evaluations
    - Helps conceptualize, plan, and communicate with others about the program
    - Uses flowcharts to help clarify key elements of a program
    - Inputs—resources that are needed to run the program
    - Educational strategies
    - Outputs—student demographics, contact hours, assignments, tests
    - Initial outcomes—changes noted in students in response to the learning activities
    - Intermediate outcomes—longer-term student outcomes
    - Ultimate outcomes—vision of what the final product should look like once students have completed the program

- Decision-Oriented Models: CIPP (Context, Input, Process, Product)
    - Provides information upon which decisions can be made, measures strengths and weaknesses of a program, identifies target populations, and identifies options
    - Uses context evaluation to identify the target population and assess their needs
    - Uses input evaluation to assess the capabilities of the system, alternative program strategies, and procedural designs useful to implement the strategy
    - Process evaluation detects defects in the design or implementation of the strategy, as well as satisfaction with the experience
    - Product evaluation reflects the outcomes and results of the program

- Fourth-Generation Models
    - "Incorporates evaluator observations, interviews, and participant evaluations to elicit views, meaning, and understanding of the stakeholders" (Bourke & Ihrke, 2009, p. 396)
    - Provides meaning, consensus, and understanding of all involved

- Accreditation Model: Evidence-Based Evaluation
    - Process used in institutions of higher learning and professional programs to determine the extent to which a program achieves its mission, goals, and outcomes
    - Focus is on ongoing self-evaluation and the achievement of outcomes to support quality improvement of the program

■  Two main organizations accredit nursing programs

   ■  National League for Nursing Accrediting Commission (NLNAC)
      (www.nlnac.org)
   ■  Commission on Collegiate Nursing Education (CCNE) (www.
      aacn.nche.edu)

## Evaluation Methods

After an evaluation model has been determined, the method(s) of evaluation
must be selected to assess the effectiveness of learning and achievement of
course and program outcomes in both their theoretical and clinical components.
Multiple methods are often used since learning is evaluated in the three domains: cognitive, affective, and psychomotor. Using a single evaluation method
does not adequately measure all three domains (see Table 4.1).

In any case, the student must be informed of the evaluation methods to be
used to assess his or her learning. Grading rubrics are one method of evaluation
that includes rating scales that are used to evaluate written work and assign a
grade. Grading rubrics are usually shared with the student before the evaluation process so the student is aware of the criteria. Grading rubrics are useful
when evaluating:

■  Tests/examinations (paper/pencil, computer)
■  Written work

   ■  Papers and essays
   ■  Portfolios
   ■  Critiques
   ■  Journals
   ■  Nursing care plans
   ■  Concept maps

■  Audiotape and videotape
■  Role-playing
■  Oral presentations
■  Simulations
■  Observations by the instructor
■  Rating scales
■  Skills checklists

Many faculty use grading rubrics to assess participation in electronic discussion boards. Rubrics range from extremely detailed to rating scales that are
more general and therefore contain some subjectivity. Table 4.2 is an example
of a grading rubric used for a journal assignment.

## Achievement Tests and Assessments

In order to ensure effective evaluation, achievement tests should be related to
the instruction given. The test questions should measure the achievement of the

| Table 4.1 | Domains and Assessment Strategies | |
|---|---|---|
| **Assessment Strategy** | **Domain of Learning Assessed** | **Uses of Assessment Strategy** |
| Papers/essays | Affective<br>Higher levels of cognitive | Demonstrates organizational skills<br>Encourages creativity<br>Improves critical thinking skills |
| Portfolios | Affective<br>Higher levels of cognitive | Measures program outcomes<br>Shows evidence of student progress in a specific class<br>Advance placement of students within courses |
| Critiques | High level cognitive<br>Affective | Active student involvement<br>Builds critical thinking skills<br>Reinforces expected standards |
| Journals | High level cognitive<br>Affective | Allows for student reflection on experiences<br>Promotes active learning<br>Assessment of student learning<br>Enhances critical thinking skills<br>Helps improve writing skills |
| Concept maps | Cognitive (all levels)<br>Affective | Visual representation of concepts and connections<br>Improves critical thinking<br>Promotes understanding of complex relationships between concepts<br>Integrates theoretical knowledge into practice |
| Audiotape | Cognitive (all levels)<br>Affective | Demonstrates communication skills<br>Demonstrates interview skills |
| Videotape | High level cognitive<br>Affective<br>Psychomotor | Review student performance of skills<br>Allows student to observe their performances<br>Reflection of the experience |
| Role playing | Cognitive<br>Affective<br>Psychomotor | Explores feelings about an experience or issue<br>Develops problem-solving skills<br>Reflects on the experience<br>Effects changes in attitude, beliefs, or values |
| Oral presentations | Cognitive<br>Affective | Improves communication skills<br>Enhances critical thinking<br>Improves organizational skills |
| Simulations | Cognitive<br>Affective<br>Psychomotor | Practice skills in a nonthreatening environment<br>Improves critical thinking skills<br>Improves prioritization of activities<br>Active learning<br>Assessment of student learning |

Adapted from *Teaching in Nursing* (3rd ed.), by D. M. Billings and J. A. Halstead, 2009. St. Louis, MO: Saunders Elsevier, p. 415.

| Table 4.2 | Example of a Rubric for Grading Journals | | | |
|---|---|---|---|---|
| Task | 1 Point | 2 Points | 3 Points | 4 Points |
| Identify goals and attainment | Goals not clearly identified. No description of attainment of goals. | Goals not clearly identified. Minimal description of attainment of goals. | Goals clearly identified. Attainment of goals mentioned, but not described completely | Goals clearly identified. Attainment of goals thoroughly discussed. |
| Score: ( /4) | | | | |
| Summary of interactions | Briefly summarized interactions with preceptor. No identification of situations encountered. | Briefly summarized interactions with preceptor. Minimal identification of situations encountered. | Summarized interactions with preceptor. Identified situations encountered. | Thoroughly summarized interactions with preceptor. Identified situations encountered. |
| Score: ( /4) | | | | |
| Analysis of significant events | No critical reflection evident in the analysis of the experience. Minimal to no description of feelings, reactions, or responses. Last journal includes little or no discussion of attainment of objectives and lessons learned. | Analysis shows minimal reflection of the experience. Minimal description of feelings, reactions, or responses. Last journal includes minimal discussion of attainment of objectives and lessons learned. | Analysis shows some critical reflection of the experience. Feelings, reactions, and responses described. Last journal includes discussion of attainment of objectives and lessons learned. | Analysis shows critical reflection of the experience. Feelings, reactions, and responses described in depth Last journal includes discussion of attainment of objectives and lessons learned. |
| Score: ( /4) | | | | |
| Submission of journals | | Journals submitted late. | | Journals submitted by due date |
| Score: ( /4) | | | | |
| Total Score: ( /16) = % | | | | |

learning outcomes and should fit the student population's learning characteristics. The results of achievement tests should be reliable and valid, and students should benefit from the test's feedback. The results should also provide faculty feedback about content areas on which they may need to put more emphasis or areas that were interpreted differently than expected (Gronlund, 1993). Achievement testing can be an effective evaluative mechanism for both student and faculty if they are developed based on sound, evaluative principles.

## Guidelines for Testing

There are three types of evaluative mechanisms used in nursing education. *Achievement tests* usually denote tests that have sound psychometric reliability; many times, these are standardized tests created by an outside vendor. *Norm-referenced tests* are those that rank a group of students. Someone gets the highest score, someone else receives the lowest, and the scores in between are compared to the shape of a "bell curve" for that evaluation. A *criterion-referenced test* is one that is closely aligned to an achievement test. The criteria are set and the score is compared to a criterion, not to other scores. The specific characteristics of each type of test are listed here (Gronlund, 1993).

### Achievement Testing

- Achievement tests should measure clearly defined learning outcomes.
  - These tests are measured in terms of student performance.
- Achievement tests should be concerned with all intended learning outcomes.
  - These tests must include outcomes based on knowledge, skill, understanding, application, and complex learning.
- Achievement tests should measure a representative sample of instructionally relevant learning skills.
  - These tests are based on sampling.
  - Instructors need to use a systematic procedure to obtain a representative sample of the test items relevant to the instruction.
  - Instructors need to prepare students for test specifications.
- Achievement tests should include the types of test items that are most appropriate for measuring the intended outcomes.
  - The tests need a means of determining if the specified performance and learning has occurred.
  - Key: select the most appropriate item type and construct it to elicit the desired response.
- Achievement tests should be based on plans for using the results.
- Achievement tests should provide scores that are relatively free from measurement errors.
  - The test should provide consistent results (it should be reliable)
  - Factors that increase the amount of error in test scores
    - Ambiguous test items

- Testing a specific skill with too few test items yields scores that are influenced by chance rather than student performance
- Essay tests are subjective
- Students' attention, effort, fatigue, and guessing on tests

### Norm-Referenced Tests

- Interpreted in relation to the ranking of students in the class
- Tell how a student's scores compare with those of his or her peers
- Provide a wide range of scores to discriminate among levels of achievement
- Focus on a broad range of learning tasks
- Feature relatively few test items per task
- Focus on student ranking
- Provide a percentile rank of students from high to low achievers
- These are commonly used in national standardized tests, such as SATs and ATIs (Gronlund, 1993; McDonald, 2007)

### Criterion-Referenced Tests

- These tests are expressed in terms of the specific knowledge and skills a student can demonstrate
- Include test items that are directly relevant to the learning outcomes regardless of the degree of difficulty
- Focus on a detailed learning domain
- Should be designed to measure the ability of a student in a particular area
- Feature a relatively large number of test items per task
- Most are teacher-made and based on course objectives
- Items provide a detailed description of student performance
- Scores are reported as the percentage correct based on preset standards
- Example: 100% of the students will correctly calculate medication dosages on the calculation exam (Gronlund, 1993; McDonald, 2007)

## Planning the Test

The first step in planning a test is to determine what type of test should be given. This decision is based on the purpose of the test. The type of test given should effectively measure the learning or capability to be measured and the desired outcome of the test. Some examples of reasons why a test may be given include:

- To determine eligibility prior to entry into a nursing program as part of the admission criteria
- To determine appropriate academic placement
- To monitor learning progress
- To determine levels of mastery of content at the end of an instruction period

# Identifying and Defining Learning Outcomes

The next step in planning a test is to identify and define intended learning outcomes. The use of Bloom's Taxonomy of Learning is one method to accomplish this step (Refer to Chapter 2 to review Bloom's Taxonomy).

- The cognitive domain addresses areas related to intellectual abilities.
- The affective domain is concerned with values and attitudes.
- The psychomotor domain addresses motor skills.
- See Table 4.3 for Bloom's Taxonomy: Affective Domain.

Achievement testing is focused primarily on the cognitive domain, with the following six main areas to consider (Gronlund, 1993):

- Knowledge (remembering previously learned material)
- Intellectual abilities and skills

    - Comprehension (grasping the meaning of material)

        - Translation (converting from one form to another)
        - Interpretation (explaining material)
        - Extrapolation (extending the meaning beyond data)

    - Application (using information in a concrete situation)
    - Analysis (breaking down material into its parts)

        - Identify the parts
        - Identify the relationships
        - Identify the organization

    - Synthesis (putting parts together to create a whole)

        - Uniqueness
        - Abstract relations

    - Evaluation (judging the value for a given purpose using specific criteria)

        - Judgment in terms of internal evidence
        - Judgment in terms of external criteria

Another method used to plan a test is to use the NCLEX-RN Test Plan (2007). Client needs are the basis of the test plan and include four major categories:

- Safe, effective care environment
- Health promotion and maintenance
- Psychosocial integrity
- Physiological integrity

Each category is assigned a percentage of the number of questions on the NCLEX-RN (see Table 4.4). Most items are concerned with the application and

| Table 4.3 | Bloom's Taxonomy—Affective Domain | |
|---|---|---|
| **Level** | **Concepts** | **Verbs Used in Writing Objectives and Learning Outcomes, With Examples** |
| Receiving | Awareness<br>Willingness to-receive<br>Control of selected attention | *Verbs*: Ask, listen, focus, attend, take part, discuss, acknowledge, hear, be open to, retain, follow, concentrate, read, do, feel<br>*Examples*: Listens to teacher or trainer; takes interest in session or learning experience; takes notes; attends; makes time for learning experience; participates passively |
| Responding | Acquiescence in responding<br>Willingness to respond<br>Satisfaction with response | *Verbs*: React, respond, seek clarification, interpret, clarify, provide other references and examples, contribute<br>*Examples*: Participate actively in group discussion, active participation in activity; show interest in outcomes; enthusiasm for action, question and probe ideas; suggest interpretations |
| Valuing | Acceptance of a value<br>Preference for a value<br>Commitment | *Verbs*: Argue, challenge, debate, refute, confront, justify, persuade, criticize<br>*Examples*: Decide worth and relevance of ideas or experiences; accept or commit to particular stance or action |
| Organization | Conceptualization of a Value<br>Organization of a value system | *Verbs*: Build, develop, formulate, defend, modify, relate, prioritize, reconcile, contrast, arrange, compare<br>*Examples*: Qualify and quantify personal views, state personal position and reasons, state beliefs |
| Characterization by a value or a value complex | General set of behaviors that characterize a person<br>Characterization of the whole person—an internal consistency | *Verbs*: Act, display, influence, solve, practice<br>*Examples*: Self-reliant; behaves consistently with personal value set |

analysis level, but the exam also includes knowledge and comprehension questions. Categories of nursing knowledge included are:

- Nursing care and caring
- Communication
- Effect of age, sex, culture, ethnicity, and religion on health needs
- Documentation

| Table 4.4 | NCLEX-RN Test Plan | |
|---|---|---|
| **Client Health Needs Tested** | | **Percentage of Test** |
| Safe, effective care environment | | |
| – Management of care | | 13–19 |
| – Safety & infection control | | 8–14 |
| Health promotion and maintenance | | 6–12 |
| Psychosocial integrity | | 6–12 |
| Physiological integrity | | |
| – Basic care/comfort | | 6–12 |
| – Pharmacological & parenteral therapies | | 13–19 |
| – Reduction of risk potential | | 13–19 |
| – Physiological adaptation | | 11–17 |

From "2007 NCLEX-RN Detailed Test Plan," by the National Council State Board of Nursing, 2007. Chicago: Author. Retrieved November 26, 2008 from http://www.ncsbn.org.

- Self-care
- Teaching-learning
- Fundamentals
- Nutrition
- Pharmacology
- Communicable diseases
- Natural and behavioral sciences.

## Determining the Types of Test Questions to Use

Once you have determined the purpose of the test and the plan to be used in its construction, the next step is to decide the types of test questions to be included. This decision is based on the objectives and outcomes for the test and can include a variety of types of questions, such as:

- Multiple choice
- True/false
- Matching
- Fill in the blank
- Essay

A table of specifications (test plan, test blueprint) should be used as the basis for developing achievement tests (see Table 4.5 for a Test Blueprint for the Nursing Process).

The following factors should be taken into consideration when developing a table of specifications:

- Matches the purpose of the test—be sure that the test is measuring a relative sample of the content and learning outcomes

| Table 4.5 | Test Blueprint: Nursing Process | | | | | |
|---|---|---|---|---|---|---|
| Content Area | Assessment | Analysis | Planning | Implementation | Evaluation | Total Number of Items |
| Cardiac % | | | | | | |
| Renal % | | | | | | |
| Endocrine % | | | | | | |
| Total number of items | | | | | | |

- Relates learning outcomes to content
- Indicates the relative weight for each area based on several factors (see Table 4.5, the Test Blueprint)
  - How much time was spent on each area during instruction? This should be the most important consideration
  - Which outcomes are most important in regards to retention and transfer value?

Another consideration that should be part of the table of specifications would be to determine the number of questions for each part of the content being tested based on the criteria listed above (see Table 4.6 for an Example of Distribution of Test Questions by Content).

## Validity and Reliability of Tests

*Validity* refers to the appropriateness, meaningfulness, and usefulness of the *inferences* from the test scores (Gronlund, 1993). A test's validity is the judgment one makes to determine if the test measured what was intended.

| Table 4.6 | Example of Distribution of Test Questions by Content | | | | |
|---|---|---|---|---|---|
| Outcomes/Content | Knowledge Terms | Facts | Comprehends Principles | Applies Principles | Total Number of Items |
| Role of nurse in decision-making | 4 | 4 | 3 | 5 | 16 |
| Osteoarthritis | 3 | 2 | 4 | 5 | 14 |
| Total # of items | 7 | 6 | 7 | 10 | 30 |

Approaches for testing validity include the following (Gronlund, 1993):

- ▓ Content-related evidence

  - ▓ How well does the test measure the intended learning outcomes?
  - ▓ Did the test feature an adequate sampling of material?
  - ▓ Was the test properly constructed, administered, and scored?

- ▓ Criterion-related evidence

  - ▓ How accurately does test performance predict future performance?
  - ▓ Can one use test performance to estimate current performance on a criterion?
  - ▓ What is the degree of relationship between the test scores and the criterion—the key element?
  - ▓ What was the correlation coefficient (r)?

    - ▓ Positive relationship—high or low scores on one measure are accompanied by high or low scores on another
    - ▓ Negative relationship—high scores on one measure are accompanied by low scores on another measure

- ▓ Construct-related evidence

  - ▓ How well can test performance be explained in terms of psychological characteristics?

*Reliability* refers to the degree of consistency of test scores. Factors that may affect reliability include insufficient length and group variability (Twigg, 2009). Reliability is measured by a correlation coefficient. The simplest method of estimating the reliability of test scores from a single administration of a test is using the Kuder-Richardson formulas (KR-20 or KR-21). The KR-20 reflects the accuracy or power of discrimination of the test (Kehoe, 1995). Three types of information are required to determine the KR: (1) the number of items in the test, (2) the mean, and (3) the standard deviation (Gronlund, 1993). The formula for the KR-20 is shown in Exhibit 4.1.

Reported reliabilities for standardized achievement tests are .90 or better for KR formulas. Reliability coefficients for classroom tests should be between .50 and .80 (1.0 is the maximum) (Kehoe, 1995).

---

**Exhibit 4.1**     **KR-21 Formula**

Reliability estimate $(KR21) = 1 - \dfrac{M(K-M)}{K(s^2)}$

K = number of items in the test
M = mean of test scores
s = standard deviation of test scores

## Factors That Lower Reliability of Test Scores (Gronlund, 1993; Kehoe, 1995)

- Too few items on the test
- Excessive numbers of very easy or very hard questions
- Inadequate testing conditions
- Items are poorly written and do not discriminate
- Scoring is subjective (remedy: prepare scoring keys and follow them carefully when scoring essay answers and performance tasks; in other words, prepare a rubric)

Exhibit 4.2 provides an example of a test statistic. Try to interpret the meaning of the statistics.

## Item Analysis

Item analysis is done to determine if tests have separated the learners from the non-learners (discrimination). Software packages can provide statistical data about the overall analysis of a test and a detailed analysis of each item. The following key concepts are necessary to consider when reviewing the item analysis on a classroom test.

- Item difficulty (P value) (Gronlund, 1993)

    - Percentage of the group who answered the item correctly
    - P = .5 (50% correct) is a good discrimination index
    - Upper limit = 1.00 (100% of students answered the question correctly)
    - Lower limit depends on the number of possible responses and probability of guessing correctly
    - If there are four options, then P = .25 is the lower limit or probability of guessing
    - See Exhibit 4.3 for a Formula for Calculating Item Difficulty

- Item Discrimination (Gronlund, 1993)
    - Differentiates between learners who knew the content from those who did not.

| Exhibit 4.2 | Sample Test Statistics | | | |
|---|---|---|---|---|
| Total Possible Points | 50 | Median Score | 40.33 | Mean Score 40.35 |
| Students in this group | 17 | | | |
| Standard Deviation | 3.53 | | | |
| Reliability Coefficient (KR20) | 0.56 | | | |
| Point Biserial | 0.18 | | | |
| Total Group | 64.71% | | | |
| Upper 27% of Group | 80.00% | | | |

- Measured by point biserial correlation (measures each student's item performance with each student's overall test performance).

  - Questions that discriminate well have point biserial correlations that are highly positive for the correct answer and negative for the distractors.
  - Learners who knew the content answered correctly, those who did not chose the distractors.
  - Indices greater than .3 are good; greater than .4 are very good.
  - Item difficulty of P = .5 shows a discrimination index that is maximized. If the index is too high or too low the index is attenuated and the item is a poor discriminator.

- Distractor Evaluation

  - Need to evaluate each distractor individually.
  - Distractors should appeal to the nonlearner.
  - Distractors that have a point biserial of zero means students did not select them and they need to be revised or replaced—students probably got the question correct by guessing.
  - Negative discriminating power occurs when more students in the lower group than in the upper group choose the correct answer. These items need to be revised or replaced.

- Compute Item Analysis

  1. Mean score—the average of all the students
  2. Median—the point at which 50% are higher and 50% are lower
  3. Standard deviation—measures the variability of test scores; the degree test scores deviate from mean

| Exhibit 4.3 | Formula for Calculating Item Difficulty | | | |
|---|---|---|---|---|

**EXAMPLE**

| ITEM 1. ALTERNATIVES | A | B* | C | D |
|---|---|---|---|---|
| Upper 10 | 0 | 6 | 3 | 1 |
| Lower 10 | 3 | 2 | 2 | 3 |

$$P = \frac{R}{T} \times 100$$

$$P = \frac{8}{20} \times 100 = 40\% \ (.40)$$

P = the percentage who answered the item correctly, R = the number who answered the item correctly, T = total number who attempted the item.

4. D value $= \dfrac{R_u - R_L}{1/2\ T}$

- D = index of discriminating power; $R_u$ = number in the upper group who answered the item correctly; $R_L$ = number in the lower group who answered the item correctly; 1/2 T = one half of the total number of students included in the item analysis.

In other words, for a multiple choice question to be discriminating it should be answered correctly by the upper 1/3 of the class and answered wrong by the lower 1/3 of the class. See Exhibit 4.4 for a Formula for Calculating Point Biserials.

Some evaluators like to purposely include one or two easy questions at the beginning of an exam to decrease students' anxiety (see Exhibit 4.5).

- Item Revision

  - Completed after item analysis
  - Revise items with the following characteristics:

    - P values that are too high or too low
    - Correct answers with low positive or negative point biserials
    - Distractors with highly positive point biserials
    - Items that correlate less than .15 with total test scores should be restructured. They are probably confusing or misleading to those taking the exam (Kehoe, 1995).

---

## Exhibit 4.4    Formula for Calculating Point Biserial

Formula for Calculating Point Biserial

| ITEM 1. ALTERNATIVES | A | B* | C | D |
|---|---|---|---|---|
| Upper 10 | 0 | 6 | 3 | 1 |
| Lower 10 | 3 | 2 | 2 | 3 |

D value $= \dfrac{R_u - R_L}{\frac{1}{2}\ T}$

$D = \dfrac{0 - 3}{10} = -0.3$ (for answer A)

$D = \dfrac{6 - 2}{10} = .40$ (for answer B)

$D = \dfrac{3 - 2}{10} = 0.1$ (for answer C)

$D = \dfrac{1 - 3}{10} = -0.2$ (for answer D)

---

**Exhibit 4.5** — **Critical Thinking Questions**

---

1. What do you do if you have a question that 100% of the class gets right?

$$\text{D value} = \frac{0 - 0}{0}$$

$$= 0 \text{ for the D value or split biserial value}$$

*Is this a discriminating question?* YES _____ NO _____

Rationale for answer: No, everyone got it correct.

2. Five out of the top third of the class chose the correct answer on an exam question; six out of the middle third, and eight out of the lower third chose the correct answer. Calculate the point biserial for this question as indicated below.

$$\text{D value} = \frac{5 - 8}{10}$$

$$= \frac{-3}{10}$$

$$= -0.3 \text{ for the D value or split bi-serial value}$$

*Is this a discriminating question?* YES _____ NO _____

Rationale for answer: The question is too difficult or unclear.

3. All students ($n = 10$) in the upper group answered an item correctly on an exam, but none of the students in the lower group got it correct.

$$D = \frac{10 - 0}{10} = 1.00$$

*Is this a discriminating question?* YES _____ NO _____

Rationale for answer: Question is too difficult and does not discriminate.

---

- The distractor was not chosen by any student. This prevents discriminating the good students from the poor students (Kehoe, 1995).
- Items that all test takers get right. These questions do not discriminate among students and should be replaced by more difficult ones.

## Outcome Evaluation

"Educational evaluation occurs while assessing the program for its quality, currency, relevance, projections into the future, and the need for possible revisions in light of these factors" (Keating, 2006, p. 260). Program evaluation encompasses all aspects of the program, including the curriculum, student satisfaction, congruency of the mission of the nursing program with that of the institution, faculty and staff qualifications, student policies and development, and resources to promote achievement of the outcomes. Accreditation of nursing programs is voluntary but encouraged, as it is a public statement attesting to the quality of the program. Several accrediting bodies oversee this process:

- State Commissions of Higher Education—the entire academic institution and programs of study are evaluated by this body
- National League for Nursing Accrediting Commission (NLNAC)—evaluates diploma, Baccalaureate, and Master's nursing programs; also LPN programs
- Commission on Collegiate Nursing Education (CCNE)—evaluates Baccalaureate, Master's and some doctoral programs

Evaluation of the nursing program is an ongoing process. Table 4.7 gives an example of a program evaluation plan.

An essential component of program evaluation is the assessment of student outcomes. This can be achieved in several ways:

- Satisfaction surveys
  - Exit interviews—conducted at the conclusion of the program, prior to graduation.
  - Employer and graduate surveys—conducted at a designated period of time, such as nine months, one year, and so on. The purpose of the survey is to determine the satisfaction of the employer with the graduate nurse's ability to function effectively within the work environment. Graduates of the program are also surveyed to determine their satisfaction with the nursing program in preparing them for the responsibilities of a graduate nurse.
- Graduation and retention rates of the program
- Standardized exam pass rates—NCLEX-RN, certification exams
- Employment opportunities

A summation of program outcomes is discussed in Exhibit 4.6.

## Evidence-Based Education

In a study examining the use of standardized computerized testing programs, the program was given for free for the first year. The second year, the students had to pay for it. Students were asked whether the testing materials were useful. Twenty-two of the students rated the materials as very or somewhat useful, 27% rated them as neutral, 27% rated them as somewhat useful or not useful. Twenty-four percent of the students did not answer the question. When examining further use of the exams ($n = 231$), 47 students thought the testing should be optional, 35 students felt the topics should be integrated into classes, 25 students believed that testing should not affect their grade, and 13 thought testing should be discontinued. The cost of the program was found to be a significant factor in deterring students from taking the exam (Richards & Stone, 2008).

# Table 4.7    Example of Program Evaluation Plan

Standard Curriculum: The curriculum prepares students to achieve the outcomes of the nursing education unit, including safe practice in contemporary health care environments

| | Process | | | | Implementation | |
| --- | --- | --- | --- | --- | --- | --- |
| Component | Where Documentation is Found | Person Responsible | Frequency of Assessment | Assessment Method(s) | Results and Analysis of Data Collection and Levels of Achievement | Actions Needed/ Not Needed |
| Curriculum flows in a logical progression | Curriculum committee minutes, class, and clinical evaluation tools | Curriculum committee chairperson | Every eight years, or when revisions occur | Comparison of curriculum elements for internal consistency | Due date | Criterion met, no action required |

From *NLNAC accreditation manual*, by the National League for Nursing Accrediting Commission, 2008. New York: Author. Retrieved November 1, 2008, from www.nlnac.org.

| Exhibit 4.6 | NLNAC Accreditation Standard 6: Outcomes |
|---|---|

Evaluation of student learning demonstrates that graduates have achieved identified competencies consistent with the institutional mission and professional standards, and that the outcomes of the nursing education unit have been achieved.

# CASE STUDIES

## Case Study 4.1

The NCLEX-RN© pass rate for first time test takers graduating from a nursing program has been 80% for the last 2 years. The program evaluation committee is charged with assessing all aspects of the nursing curriculum, including admission and progression criteria, course evaluations, and scores on standardized and classroom tests. The current admission policy into the nursing program is congruent with the university's admission policies. They include the following criteria: SAT scores of 980 or better; upper half of graduating class; minimum GPA of 2.0. Once enrolled in the nursing major, students must maintain a minimum cumulative GPA of 2.5, and grades of C or better (75%) in the nursing and science courses. At this university students must meet admission and progression requirements established by the university, but individual programs may require more stringent policies for the major. As a member of the admission and progression committee in the nursing department, what recommendations would you make regarding admission into the nursing major? What recommendations would you make regarding progression in the nursing major through each level? What, if any, changes would you make relative to grading criteria, teacher-made tests, and the use of standardized achievement tests? Develop a program evaluation plan based on your recommendations.

## Case Study 4.2

You are a member of the admission, progression, and graduation committee. There is a concern regarding declining pass rates on the NCLEX-RN exam. The committee has been charged with reviewing and revising the admission and progression standards. What areas would you consider to be priorities to address as part of the revision of the standards in order to improve NCLEX-RN pass rates?

## Practice Questions

1. The Program Evaluation committee of the nursing program is reviewing the program evaluation data. The nursing program has established an 86% pass rate as the benchmark for graduates taking the NCLEX-RN exam for the

first time. This goal has not been met for the past three years. Which of the following recommendations would be a priority for the committee to make?

A. Increase the passing grade for each nursing course to 83%.
B. Require a minimum GPA of 3.0 in all natural science and nursing courses.
C. Lower the NCLEX-RN pass rate benchmark for first-time takers to 78%.
D. Institute a pre-RN assessment test with a minimum benchmark for admission into the nursing program.

2. A clinical instructor is preparing to write the summative evaluation for the students in her clinical group. She believes in the Constructivist philosophy of evaluation. Therefore, when completing the evaluation, she will do which of the following?

A. Determine if the objectives of the course have been met.
B. Compare the students to other students to determine each student's level of development.
C. Seek input from clinical staff regarding each student's clinical performance.
D. Assign a grade of pass/fail for the clinical performance.

3. The nursing curriculum committee is revising the curriculum to be more congruent with changes in health care delivery. The most important consideration of the committee should be which of the following?

A. Be sure the new curriculum is aligned with the mission and philosophy of the governing institution.
B. Develop curriculum objectives and program outcomes.
C. Establish benchmarks for first time pass rates on the NCLEX-RN exam.
D. Require a standardized exit exam with a benchmark passing rate of 85%.

4. A nurse educator is reviewing the item analysis on a course test for a multiple-choice question. The following statistics were calculated for this item:

| Point Biserial = –0.27 | Correct answer = B | | Total group = 88.24% | |
|---|---|---|---|---|
| Distractor Analysis: | A | B | C | D |
| Pt-Biserial: | 0.27 | –0.27 | 0.00 | 0.00 |
| Frequency: | 12% | 88% | 0% | 0% |

The educator realizes the cause for this frequency distribution is:

A. The distractors were not clear.
B. The distractors were too hard for students to choose.
C. Students who scored lower on the exam got the item correct.
D. Students who knew the content answered the item correctly.

5. The following statistics were calculated on a multiple-choice question on an exam:

| Point Biserial = 0.61 | Correct answer = C | | Total group = 76.47% | |
|---|---|---|---|---|
| Distractor Analysis: | A | B | C | D |
| Pt-Biserial: | –0.59 | 0.00 | 0.61 | –0.24 |
| Frequency: | 6% | 0% | 88% | 6% |

The reason for this frequency distribution is:
A. Students who scored lower on the exam got the item correct.
B. The distractors were not clear.
C. This item has been used on previous exams.
D. Students who scored higher on the exam got the item correct.

6. The item analysis revealed the following data for a multiple-choice question:

| Point Biserial = 0.19 | Correct answer = D | | Total group = 5.88% | |
|---|---|---|---|---|
| Distractor Analysis: | A | B | C | D |
| Pt-Biserial: | −0.25 | 0.39 | −0.35 | 0.19 |
| Frequency: | 41% | 41% | 12% | 6% |

Based on these statistics, the professor should do which of the following when using this item on future exams:
A. Nothing, as the upper third of the class answered the item correctly
B. Revise distractor A
C. Revise distractor B
D. Revise distractor C

7. An item analysis report for a multiple-choice exam revealed that the KR20 was 0.56. Based on this statistic, which of the following interpretations can be made regarding this exam?
A. The exam is reliable in measuring student knowledge of the material.
B. There are too few items on the exam.
C. The items are poorly written and do not discriminate.
D. There is an excess of very easy questions.

8. A professor administered a multiple-choice exam and performed an item analysis, which revealed the following data:

| Point Biserial = 0.56 | Correct answer = A | | Total group = 52.94% | |
|---|---|---|---|---|
| Distractor Analysis: | A | B | C | D |
| Pt-Biserial: | 0.56 | −0.31 | −0.44 | 0.02 |
| Frequency: | 52% | 18% | 18% | 12% |

The likely cause for this frequency distribution is:
A. The distractors are too hard.
B. Students who scored highest on the exam got the item correct.
C. The distractors are too easy.
D. Students guessed the answer to this question.

9. The following statistics were obtained in an item analysis for a multiple-choice exam:

| Point Biserial = 0.00 | Correct answer = C | | Total group = 100% | |
|---|---|---|---|---|
| Distractor Analysis: | A | B | C | D |
| Pt-Biserial: | 0.00 | 0.00 | 0.00 | 0.00 |
| Frequency: | 0% | 0% | 100% | 0% |

What action should be taken based on this data?
A. No action is needed as all students answered the question correctly.
B. Revise distractor C.
C. Add another distractor to the choices.
D. Rewrite all of the distractors.

10. Which of the following activities would be the best strategy to engage the visual learner at the cognitive and affective levels?
A. Audiotaping a lecture
B. Writing a case study
C. Developing a concept map
D. Writing an essay

# References

Angelo, T. A. (1993). Teacher's dozen: Fourteen general, research-based principles for improving higher learning in our classrooms. Retrieved December 12, 2008, from http://ir.atu.edu/Retention_Info/retentionother/Thomas_Angelo's_14_Principles.pdf

Billings, D., & Halstead, J. A. (1999). *Teaching in nursing* (3rd ed.). St. Louis, MO: Saunders Elsevier.

Bourke, M. P., & Ihrke, B. A. (2009). The evaluation process: An overview. In D. M. Billings & J. A. Halstead (Eds.), *Teaching in nursing* (3rd ed., pp. 443–464). St. Louis, MO: Saunders Elsevier.

Commission on Collegiate Nursing Education. (2008). *Procedures for accreditation of baccalaureate and graduate degree nursing programs.* Washington, DC: Author. Retrieved December 1, 2008, from http://www.aacn.nche.edu

dela Cruz, F., & Klakovich, M. (2008, September 19). *Transitioning second career students to nursing.* Paper presented at the meeting of the National League for Nursing Educational Summit, San Antonio, TX.

Farnsworth, J., & Springer, P. (2006). Background checks for nursing students: What are schools doing? *Nursing Education Perspectives, 27*(3), 48–53.

Gronlund, N. E. (1993). *How to make achievement tests and assessments* (5th ed.). Boston: Allyn and Bacon.

Keating, S. B. (2006). *Curriculum development and evaluation in nursing.* Philadelphia: Lippincott Williams & Wilkins.

Kehoe, J. (1995). Basic item analysis for multiple-choice tests. *Practical Assessment, Research & Evaluation, 4*(10). Retrieved December 2, 2008, from http://PAREonline.net/getvn.asp?v=4&n=10

Mahara, M. S. (1998). A perspective on clinical evaluation in nursing education. *Journal of Advanced Nursing, 28*(6), 1339–1346.

McDonald, M. E. (2007). *The nurse educator's guide to assessing learning outcomes* (2nd ed.). Boston: Jones and Bartlett Publishers.

National Council of State Boards of Nursing. (2007). 2007 NCLEX-RN Detailed test plan. Chicago: Author. Retrieved November 26, 2008 from http://www.ncsbn.org

National League for Nursing. (2005). *Core competencies of nurse educators with task statements.* New York: Author. Retrieved November 1, 2008, from www.nln.org

National League for Nursing Accrediting Commission. (2008). *NLNAC accreditation manual.* New York: Author. Retrieved November 1, 2008, from www.nlnac.org

Newton, S. E., & Moore, G. (2007). Undergraduate grade point average and graduate record examination scores: The experience of one graduate nursing program. *Nursing Education Perspectives, 28*(6), 327–331.

O'Connor, A. B. (2006). *Clinical instruction and evaluation: A teaching resource* (2nd ed.). Boston: Jones and Bartlett Publishers.

Orchard, C. (1994). Management of clinical failure in Canadian nursing programs. *Western Journal of Nursing Research, 16*(3), 317–331.

Richards, E. A., & Stone, C. L. (2008). Student evaluation of a standardized comprehensive testing program. *Nursing Education Perspectives, 29*(6), 363–365.

Sauter, M. K., Johnson, D. R., & Gillespie, N. N. (2009). Educational program evaluation. In D. M. Billings & J. A. Halstead (Eds.), *Teaching in nursing* (3rd ed., pp. 467–509). St. Louis, MO: Saunders Elsevier.

Sayles, S., Shelton, D., & Powell, H. (2003). Predictors of success in nursing education. *The ABNF Journal,* November/December, 116–120.

Twigg, P. (2009). Developing and using classroom tests. In D. M. Billings & J. A. Halstead (Eds.), *Teaching in nursing* (3rd ed., pp. 429–448). St. Louis, MO: Saunders Elsevier.

Yin, T., & Burger, C. (2003). Predictors of NCLEX-RN success of Associate degree nursing graduates. *Nurse Educator, 28,* 232–236.

# Curriculum Design and Evaluation of Program Outcomes, Clinical Teaching, and Learning

Marylou K. McHugh

*The materials of instruction should be selected and organized with a view to giving the learner that development most helpful in meeting and controlling life experiences*

— Decker F. Walker and Jonas F. Soltis, *Curriculum and Aims*

**NLN Core Competency IV: Participate in Curriculum Design and Evaluation of Program Outcomes**

Nurse educators are responsible for formulating program outcomes and designing curricula that reflect contemporary health care trends and prepare graduates to function effectively in the health care environment (National League for Nursing [NLN], 2005, p. 19).

**Learning Outcomes**

■ Discuss leadership and change behaviors that assist in curriculum development.
■ Explain the process of curriculum development.

■ Analyze evaluation methods appropriate to measuring program outcomes.
■ Evaluate teaching methods/strategies for classroom and clinical teaching.

## Introduction

Curriculum development can be the most creative and satisfying part of the educational process. It is dynamic and vibrant, but also demanding of the educator's time. In today's educational environment, with so much content added to the need for thoughtful practice with an emphasis on higher level thinking, the educator is challenged even more than ever.

Curriculum is a living entity and must be reviewed regularly and renewed for its relevance to the environment in which it exists. Faculty need to consider the environmental and human factors that influence the curriculum. These factors are called "the frame" and are classified as either internal or external factors (Keating, 2006).

External frame factors consist of the elements of the environment that are outside of the parent institution that influence the curriculum. All of these elements must be considered when developing a curriculum. External frame factors include the following issues and prompt the following questions:

### Financial Support

■ How will the program be financed? Are there resources available for the latest technology?
■ Does the institution have available room for the program's needs?

### Regulations and Accreditation

■ What state regulations need be considered?
■ Will the program apply for national accreditation?
■ Are there resources available to assist in these efforts?
■ How will the program meet professional standards?

### Nursing Profession

■ Are there nursing leaders and staff nurses who will support the program and act as mentors?
■ Are the professionals active and interested in the education of future nurses?

### Need for the Program

■ Does the community really need the program?
■ Is there adequate interest in the program?
■ What are the employment possibilities for the graduates?

### Demographics

■ What are the age ranges and age groups, predicted population changes, ethnic and cultural groups, and typical socioeconomic status of the community?

### Political Climate and the Body Politic

- Who are the individuals who exert influence within the community?
- Who are the players and are they supportive of the program?

### Health Care System and Health Needs of the Populace

- What are the major health care systems in the area?
- Can they be utilized for clinical experiences?
- What are the major health care problems?

### Characteristics of the Academic Setting

- What are the characteristics of the setting?
- Is it a private liberal arts college or a major research university?
- How will these characteristics inform the program?

Internal frame factors refer to those elements that are internal to the institution and inform the program. All of these elements must be considered when developing the curriculum. Internal frame factors and clarifying questions include (Keating, 2006):

### Potential Faculty and Student Characteristics

- Are there enough available, experienced faculty who have expertise in the various curriculum areas?
- What is the quantity and quality of the potential student body?

### Description and Organization Structure of the Parent Institution

- What is the quality of the physical campus and its buildings?
- What is the role of the nursing program in the institution?

### Resources Within the Institution and the Nursing Program

- Who will develop the business plan that focuses resources for program support?
- Are there endowments, financial aid programs, and/or governmental and private grants available to the program?
- Are there appropriate support services for students and faculty such as advising, academic help, library services, technology support, research help?

### Internal Economic Situation and its Influence on the Curriculum

- Is the economic status of the parent institution sound?
- Does the administration support the goals of the nursing program?

### Mission or Purpose, Philosophy, and Goals of the Parent Institution

- How will the three areas of institutional focus—research, service, and teaching—inform the nursing program and which will be prominent?
- Will there be some attempt at balance?

## Critical Thinking Questions

Have you carefully assessed your program in light of the above requirements that will impinge on curriculum development and the success of the program? Can you identify those external and internal factors that will be most influential in your curriculum development?

## Leading the Program

In any major academic endeavor, such as curriculum development, deciding on leadership is an important part of the process. What defines leadership? Where does the leader come from? Who should lead? What are the qualities that the leader will need? Leadership is the process of showing the way by going in advance, by directing the performance or activities of a group (American Heritage Dictionary, 1970). The leader may be the Dean in a small school or department of nursing. In a bigger institution, the leader may be a seasoned faculty member with some prior experience in curriculum development. Leaders may emerge from the group or may be appointed by the Dean.

A leader should possess knowledge of both the content and process of curriculum development, and a caring and compassionate attitude (Yoder-Wise, 1995). Leaders emerge in the following ways:

- *Emergent leadership*—The members of the group view the leader as someone who is knowledgeable and trustworthy; they recognize and accept the leader's influence to lead.
- *Imposed or organizational leadership*—The leader is appointed by someone outside the group. If the group members do not have confidence in the appointed leader's abilities, they may not perform to their highest potential.

Wiles and Bondi (1998) have identified 19 roles that a curriculum leader needs to fulfill:

- Expert
- Confronter
- Instructor
- Counselor
- Trainer
- Advisor
- Retriever
- Observer
- Referrer
- Data collector

- Linker
- Analyzer
- Demonstrator
- Diagnostician
- Modeler
- Designer
- Advocate
- Manager
- Evaluator

Five practices associated with exceptional leadership are (Huber, 2000):

- Challenging the process by searching for opportunities, experimenting, and taking risks.
- Inspiring a shared vision by envisioning the future and enlisting the support of others.
- Enabling others to act by fostering collaboration and strengthening others.
- Modeling the way by setting an example and planning small successes.
- Encouraging the heart by recognizing contributions and celebrating accomplishments.

Types of Leaders are described in Table 5.1 and leadership styles are depicted in Figure 5.1.

## Critical Thinking Question

Which leadership style have you seen in your nurse educator experience?

While the transformation leadership approach is often highly effective, there is no one "right" way to lead or manage that suits all situations. To choose the most effective approach for you, you must consider:

- The skill levels and experience of the members of your team
- The work involved (routine or new and creative)
- The organizational environment (stable or radically changing, conservative or adventurous)
- You own preferred or natural style

A good leader will find him or herself switching instinctively between styles according to the people and work with which they are dealing. This is often referred to as "situational leadership." Power is shared in participative leadership; is in the hands of the leader in autocratic leadership, and is left to group members in the free-rein or *laissez-faire* style of leadership.

| Table 5.1 | Leadership Styles and Associated Characteristics |
|---|---|
| **Leadership Style** | **Leadership Characteristics** |
| Democratic or Participative | ■ Invites members of the team to contribute to the decision-making process.<br>■ May make the final decision, but uses good people skills.<br>■ Team members have some control over their destiny.<br>■ May take more time than other leadership styles, but is usually more satisfying to the entire team. |
| Autocratic | ■ This is an extreme form of transactional leadership.<br>■ A leader exerts high levels of power over the team.<br>■ Team members are provided few opportunities for making suggestions.<br>■ Most people tend to resent this style; it may produce a high level of absenteeism and turnover. |
| *Laissez-faire* or Free Rein | ■ This leader leaves the work to the team.<br>■ It can be effective if the leader monitors and communicates regularly.<br>■ To work, the team must be experienced and self-starting.<br>■ The lack of control can also hinder the process. |
| Bureaucratic leadership | ■ This leader works "by the book."<br>■ Can be appropriate for serious issues involving safety.<br>■ The inflexibility and high levels of control can demoralize the team.<br>■ Can produce organizational inflexibility. |
| Charismatic | ■ This leadership style is very energetic and enthusiastic.<br>■ May focus more on themselves than the team.<br>■ This leadership style can produce over-dependency on the leader and the project may not be completed if the leader leaves. |
| Task-oriented | ■ This leadership style focuses only on getting the job done and is autocratic.<br>■ The leader defines the work and the roles required.<br>■ The leader puts structures in place, plans, organizes, and monitors.<br>■ There are difficulties in motivating and retaining staff. |
| People-oriented | ■ This style of leadership style is totally focused on organizing, supporting, and developing the team.<br>■ It is a participative style and leads to good teamwork and creative collaboration.<br>■ If extreme, it can lead to the failure to achieve the team's goals. |

*(Continued)*

| Table 5.1 | Leadership Styles and Associated Characteristics (Continued) |
|---|---|
| Transactional | ■ This leadership style asks team members to agree to obey their leader totally.<br>■ The "transaction" is what the organization pays the team members in return for their effort.<br>■ The leader has the right to "punish" team members if their work doesn't meet the pre-determined standard.<br>■ A transactional leader may "manage by exception," whereby, rather than rewarding better work, they take corrective action if it is required.<br>■ This has serious limitations for knowledge-based or creative work. |
| Transformational | ■ This leadership style inspires the team with a shared vision of the future.<br>■ They are highly visible, and spend a lot of time communicating.<br>■ They delegate responsibility amongst their teams.<br>■ They have enthusiasm, but need to be supported by "detail people." |

Adapted with permission from Mind Tools. Retrieved April 2, 2009, from http://www.mindtools.com/pages/artoc;e/newLDC_84.htm

**5.1** Leadership styles.

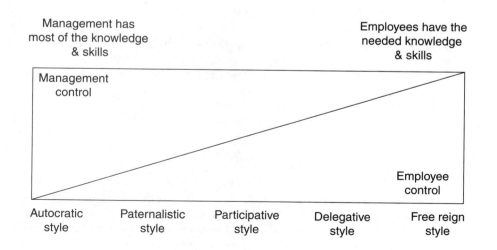

## Responsibilities of Faculty in Curriculum Development

While the leader is responsible for guiding the faculty through the curriculum process, individual faculty members have their own set of responsibilities. Many nursing leaders believe that faculty "own" the curriculum because of their expertise in content, along with a good sense of the practice world. Because of the concept of academic freedom, faculty members may investigate new theories and ideas and express opinions in the classroom that are relevant to the course being taught (Finke, 2009). This does not mean that faculty members may develop course content in isolation; rather, they must work together to develop the plan and then follow the plan they have developed. Curriculum must build in a structured way that enables the student to incorporate the art, science, and practice of nursing in a coherent manner. Faculty must strive to ensure that the program outcomes are achieved. The curriculum must also meet the requirements of both the State Board of Nursing and external accrediting bodies.

Faculty responsibilities include:

- Develop policies and procedures that affect student and faculty conduct and the curriculum;
- Advise administration and students on educational issues;
- Participate in administrative actions that affect the institution and community;
- Ensure that content and learning experiences are sequenced toward educational outcomes;
- Collect and analyze relevant information pertaining to the need for curriculum development and revision;
- Prepare graduates to function in the changing and complex health care environment; and
- Develop strategies to facilitate the exchange of ideas and decision making relevant to curriculum development and revisions (Johnson, as cited in Keating, 2006, p. 37).

There are certain attributes related to academic freedom that include the following three aspects, as set forth by the American Association of University Professors (AAUP, 1940/1970). These include:

1. Teachers are entitled to full freedom in research and in the publication of the results, subject to the adequate performance of their other academic duties; but research for pecuniary return should be based upon an understanding with the authorities of the institution.
2. Teachers are entitled to freedom in the classroom in discussing their subject, but they should be careful not to introduce into their teaching controversial matter which has no relation to their subject. Limitations of academic freedom because of religious or other aims of the institution should be clearly stated in writing at the time of the appointment.
3. College and university teachers are citizens, members of a learned profession, and officers of an educational institution. When they speak or write as citizens, they should be free from institutional censorship or discipline, but their special position in the community imposes special obligations. As scholars and educational officers, they should remember that the public

may judge their profession and their institution by their utterances. Hence they should at all times be accurate, should exercise appropriate restraint, should show respect for the opinions of others, and should make every effort to indicate that they are not speaking for the institution.

There are many factors that faculty have to consider in curriculum design; some of these are similar considerations to the total program design as mentioned previously. These factors include:

- Institutional philosophy and mission, which includes:
  1. The institution's reason for being with outcome goals;
  2. The program's philosophy and mission must reflect that of the parent institutions; and
  3. It provides a belief and value base for the curricular structure and content (Leddy, in Moyer & Wittmann-Price, 2007).

- Organizing framework
  1. The curriculum framework provides a way for faculty to conceptualize and organize knowledge, skills, values, and beliefs that are critical to the delivery of a coherent curriculum; and
  2. It facilitates the sequencing and prioritizing of knowledge in a way that is logical and internally consistent (Finke, 2009).

- Current nursing and health care trends
  1. Faculty should consider the economic and political issues that influence health care issues;
  2. Issues such as bio-terrorism, genetics, interdisciplinary education, an aging population, and the use of technology such as SIM people are important.

- Community and societal needs
  1. Changes in demographics such as ageism, sexism, and racism are pertinent topics for inclusion.
  2. The need for primary care practitioners and health educators in community settings.

- Educational principles
- Active teaching strategies for both traditional and nontraditional students should be considered
- Discussion about various educational theories should preclude the actual curriculum plan.
- Theory and research
  1. Evidence-based practice (EBP) is a current mandate; and
  2. The theory and research supporting all procedures is a priority.

- Use of technology
  1. PDAs, SIM people, and Standardized Patients (SP) are a part of health care education; and
  2. Faculty needs to discuss their integration into the curriculum (adapted from Keating, 2006, p. 165 and Leddy, 2007).

There are also accrediting body standards that need to be incorporated into curriculum design, such as the NLNAC standards 1, 4.1, 4.4, and 4.6.

- NLNAC Standard 1: The nursing education unit's mission reflects the governing organization's core values and is congruent with its strategic goals and objectives.
- NLNAC Standard 4.1: The curriculum incorporates established professional standards, guidelines, and competencies.
- NLNAC Standard 4.4: The curriculum includes cultural, ethnic, and socially diverse concepts and may also include experiences from regional, national, or global perspectives.
- NLNAC Standard 4.6: The curriculum and instructional processes reflect educational theory (National League for Nursing Accrediting Commission, 2008).

## Theoretical and Conceptual Frameworks

After completing the first step toward curriculum development, the careful review of the mission statement of both the parent institution and the nursing unit, the next step is for faculty to begin to identify the organizing framework to be used as the model for building the curriculum. All nursing programs are based on some sort of model, whether the faculty recognizes it or not (Barnum, 1998). There are many models to choose from. Remember, the framework selected for use will eventually provide students the basis for the conceptualization of their profession. It should be clear and practical, and faculty must be consistent in the way they use it. The basic curriculum models and their characteristics include:

### Curriculum Model

- Students learn the disciplines inherent to the profession
- The model may take varied forms, such as medical models
- Courses include Medical Surgical Nursing, Pediatric Nursing, Psych Mental Health Nursing, and so on

### Integrated Model

- This model addresses problems such as circulatory, respiratory, and orthopedic care; and
- Addresses the nursing care of patients at all developmental levels (infancy, childhood, adolescence, adulthood, the elderly).

### Discipline or Nursing Theorist Model

- This model is informed by a conceptual model of nursing (Levine, Orem, Neuman, or Roy)
- It may also be designed by the faculty from an intuited image of nursing (Barnum, 1998)
- The courses are specifically designed to the model (e.g., if using Levine, courses would include Problems of Conservation of Energy, Problems of Conservation of Structural Integrity, etc.).

### Deconstructed or Emancipator Curriculum Model

- ■ A deconstructed curriculum focuses on teaching thinking (Ironsides, 2004)
- ■ The emphasis is on thinking about content, not the content itself

Courses in the Curriculum Model would be very traditional. They would treat each area separately with courses such as Care of Fundamentals of Nursing, Care of the Adult I, II, and III, Pediatric Nursing, and so on. The nursing process steps, assessment, diagnosis, planning, implementation, and evaluation, would be integrated into each traditional course.

In contrast, courses in the Integrated Model would be more integrated throughout the curriculum. Examples of course titles would include Circulatory Problems Across the Life Cycle or Care of the Infant—which would then include all of the health-illness issues associated with that topic. Many educators feel that content is often lost in this kind of model, yet for some programs this model works extremely well. Table 5.2 illustrates a curriculum grid for incorporating the nursing health-illness concerns into the Integrated Model approach.

Courses in the Discipline Model are integrated into the concepts of the theory used. Table 5.3 illustrates how a nursing process may be integrated into the Dorothea Orem Theoretical Model for patients who need wholly compensatory care.

## Critical Thinking Question

What kind of curriculum model do you feel is most appropriate for your unit, faculty, and students and why?

| Table 5.2 | Integrated Model Cross Gridding Nursing Process and the Nursing Problems | | | | | |
|---|---|---|---|---|---|---|
| | Dominant: Nursing Problems Components | | | | | |
| Secondary Developmental Levels | Circulatory Health to Illness | Respiratory Health to Illness | Neurologic Health to Illness | Endocrine Health to Illness | Gastro-intestinal Health to Illness | Renal Health to Illness |
| Infancy | | | | | | |
| Childhood | | | | | | |
| Young Adult | | | | | | |
| Mid-Adult | | | | | | |
| Elderly | | | | | | |

| Table 5.3 | Discipline Model Cross Gridding Nursing Process and the Dorothea Orem System | | |
|---|---|---|---|
| Secondary Steps of the Nursing Process | Wholly Compensatory System | Partly Compensatory System | Supportive Educative System |
| Assessment | | | |
| Diagnosis | | | |
| Planning | | | |
| Intervention | | | |
| Evaluation | | | |

## Program Goals, Objectives, and Outcomes

The next stage of curriculum development is to identify the program goals, outcomes, and terminal objectives of the program. The science of writing objectives has been discussed in Chapter 2. This section discusses how to articulate a program's outcomes and develop the objectives for each level of learning. These are called "level objectives" and are used to guide the shaping of course selection and content throughout the years (or levels) in which the students progress. These statements must be specific and reflect the institution's and the program's mission statements. Faculty should discuss the following questions:

1. What exactly should the graduating students look like?
2. What characteristics and competencies do they need to posses upon completion of the program?

The curriculum has moved from one that is politically correct to one that is theoretically pluralistic; to incorporate caring and humanitarianism as core values rather than the dominations of technology; and the centrality of the student-teacher relationship over esoteric scholarship. (National League for Nursing, 1993, p. 11)

The development of specific program outcomes and goal objectives will flow from the answers derived from the discussion of these two pertinent and important questions. Leveling a program is an important concept in curriculum development; it orchestrates where to place course materials and what can be expected from students in the clinical area.

## Level Objectives

The next task pertaining to leveling and course placement is to develop level objectives that delineate what skills the student will need to develop if he or she is to achieve the program outcomes. Level objectives are meant to guide course design while feeding into the program outcomes.

Level objectives can be teased out to reflect specific program objectives, course objectives, and clinical objectives. Table 5.4 illustrates how program, course, and clinical objectives for each level lead to the final outcomes of a program.

> Program and level objectives for the program, which reflect program outcomes and plan for the sequential development of the knowledge and competencies necessary to achieve those outcomes, address the same core competencies, but at different levels of sophistication and with different populations. The related course objectives mirror the program and level objectives, but express how the objective is achieved within the content and related clinical experiences students cover in the course (O'Connor, 2006, p. 313).

- Level One: Students begin to identify the ethical issues that may affect the care of their patients;
- Level Two: The students, building on level one, apply these concepts;
- Level Three: Students are required to analyze the effects of the legal-ethical system on the care of patients, families, and communities; and
- By the end of the program, students are expected to be able to integrate these concepts into their patient care.

Based on the program outcomes and the level objectives, faculty will develop courses that will lead to the students' achievement of the goals. Competencies at the course level are much more specific and lead the faculty to prepare content, learning activities, and clinical experiences.

## Baccalaureate Outcomes of the AACN

In October 2008, the American Association of Colleges of Nursing (AACN) identified outcomes for the Baccalaureate prepared nurse that faculty should consider when planning their curricula. The outcomes directly from the AACN (2008, p. 3) include:

1. Conduct comprehensive and focused physical, behavioral, psychological, spiritual, socioeconomic, and environmental assessments of health and illness parameters in patients using developmentally and culturally appropriate approaches.
2. Recognize the relationship of genetics and genomics to health, prevention, screening, diagnostics, prognostics, selection of treatment, and the monitoring of treatment effectiveness using a constructed pedigree from collected family history information as well as standardized symbols and terminology.
3. Implement holistic, patient-centered care that reflects an understanding of human growth and development, pathophysiology, pharmacology, medical management, and nursing management across the health/illness continuum, across the lifespan, and in all health care settings.
4. Communicate effectively with all members of the health care team, including the patient and the patient's support network.

| Table 5.4 | Leveling Objectives | | |
|---|---|---|---|
| **Level One** | **Level Two** | **Level Three** | **Level Four** |
| PROGRAM OBJECTIVES | | | |
| Identify legal and ethical issues that affect the professional nurse's delivery of care to patients and their families. | Apply ethical and legal concepts to the care of patients and their families. | Analyze the effect of legal and ethical issues to the care of patients, families, and communities. | Integrates ethical/legal concepts and principles, the Code of Ethics for Nurses, and professional standards into practice within professional, academic, and community settings. |
| COURSE OBJECTIVES | | | |
| Discuss the content inherent in the ANA's Code of Ethics for Nurses. | Apply legal/ethical content to case studies involving patients and families. | Develop care plans based on criteria found in the Standards of Practice and the Code for Nurses. | Compare and contrast the appropriate Standards of Practice and Code of Ethics to various practice situations. |
| CLINICAL OBJECTIVE | | | |
| Using the Code of Ethics for Nurses, identify one issue that has impinged on your nursing care of a patient and/or their family. | Apply legal/ethical principles in caring for your patient and family. | Analyze the effects of HIPPA on the care of your patient and family. | Consciously practice using the Code of Ethics for Nurses and the appropriate Standards of Practice when caring for patients, families or communities. |

5. Deliver compassionate, patient-centered, evidence-based care that respects patient and family preferences.
6. Implement patient and family care around the resolution of end of life and palliative care issues, such as symptom management, support of rituals, and respect for patient and family preferences.
7. Provide appropriate patient teaching that reflects developmental stage, age, culture, spirituality, patient preferences, and health literacy considerations to foster patient engagement in their care.

8.  Implement evidence-based nursing interventions as appropriate for managing the acute and chronic care of patients and promoting health across the lifespan.
9.  Monitor client outcomes to evaluate the effectiveness of psychobiological interventions.
10. Facilitate patient-centered transitions of care, including discharge planning and ensuring the caregiver's knowledge of care requirements to promote safe care.
11. Provide nursing care based on evidence that contributes to safe and high quality patient outcomes within health care microsystems.
12. Create a safe care environment that results in high quality patient outcomes.
13. Revise the plan of care based on an ongoing evaluation of patient outcomes.
14. Demonstrate clinical judgment and accountability for patient outcomes when delegating to and supervising other members of the health care team.
15. Manage care to maximize health, independence, and quality of life for a group of individuals that approximates a beginning practitioner's workload.
16. Demonstrate the application of psychomotor skills for the efficient, safe, and compassionate delivery of patient care.
17. Develop a beginning understanding of complementary and alternative modalities and their roles in health care.
18. Develop an awareness of patients' and health care professionals' spiritual beliefs and values and how those beliefs and values impact health care.
19. Manage the interaction of multiple functional problems affecting patients across the lifespan, including common geriatric syndromes.
20. Understand one's role and participation in emergency preparedness and disaster response with an awareness of environmental factors and the risks they pose to oneself and patients.
21. Engage in caring and healing techniques that promote a therapeutic nurse-patient relationship.
22. Demonstrate tolerance for the ambiguity and unpredictability of the world and its effect on the health care systems as related to nursing practice.

## Changing or Revising the Curriculum

Changing an existing curriculum is sometimes more difficult than developing a curriculum from scratch because faculty have a history with the outgoing curriculum. A contemplated change process must be used in order to change an existing curriculum effectively. When leaders or managers are planning to manage change, there are five key principles that need to be kept in mind:

- Different people react differently to change.
- Everyone has fundamental needs that must be met.
- Change often involves a loss, and people go through the "loss curve."
- Expectations need to be managed realistically.

- Fears have to be dealt with.
- There should be a good reason for the change.

Here are some tips for applying the above principles when managing change:

- Give people information—be open and honest about the facts, but don't give in to overly optimistic speculation. Meet people's openness needs, but in a way that does not set unrealistic expectations.
- For large groups, produce a communication strategy that ensures information is disseminated efficiently and comprehensively to everyone (don't let the grapevine take over). Tell everyone at the same time. However, follow this up with individual interviews to produce a personal strategy for dealing with the change. This helps to recognize and deal appropriately with the individual reactions to change.
- Give people choices to make, and be honest about the possible consequences of those choices. Meet their control and inclusion needs.
- Give people time to express their views and support their decision-making. Provide coaching, counseling, or information as appropriate, to help them through the loss curve.
- Where the change involves a loss, identify what will or might replace that loss—loss is easier to cope with if there is something to replace it. This will help assuage potential fears.
- Where it is possible to do so, give individuals the opportunity to express their concerns and provide reassurances—this also to helps to assuage potential fears.
- Maintain good management practices, such as making time for informal discussions and feedback. Even though the pressure might seem that it is reasonable to let such things slip, during difficult change such practices are even more important (Team Technology, 2008).

Treat change as a project. Do this by applying all the rigors of project management to the change process: produce plans, allocate resources, appoint a steering board and/or project sponsor, etc. The five principles listed above should form part of the project objectives (Team Technology, 2008).

## First-Order and Second-Order Changes

- First-order change does not challenge or contradict the established context of an organization. This type of change does not usually threaten people, either personally or collectively.
- The deeper changes that frustrate leaders and threaten followers are planned second-order changes. These changes intentionally challenge widely-shared assumptions, disintegrate the context of "organization," and, in general, reframe the social system. This, in turn, generates wide-

spread ambiguity, discontinuity, anxiety, frustration, confusion, paranoia, cynicism and anger as well as temporary dysfunction.

## Change Theory

The varieties of change theories often used in nursing are reviewed in Chapter 7. In order to provide a theoretical example that could be used in changing a curriculum, Lewin's force-field analysis model will be used to illustrate elements of change and resistance to change.

According to this model, pressing for change tends to threaten stability and thus increases the power of forces maintaining the system. Therefore, the most effective way to bring about change is to *reduce the forces of resistance*. The major concepts of the model are outlined below (Wirth, 2004).

A force field relates to all the behaviors of a group in its environment during a given period of time.

- Driving forces—The past, present, and future elements, along with hopes, aspirations, and emotional investments that tend to affect a social event in a positive direction.
- Restraining forces—The past, present, and future elements, along with hopes, aspirations, and emotional investments that tend to affect a social event in a negative direction.
- Status quo—A dynamic equilibrium composed of a balance between the driving and restraining forces.
- Motivators—The initial stimuli that convinces the concerned parties there is a need for change.
- Confirmation of non-accomplishment—Information that confirms the fact that the desired job is not being accomplished.
- Confirmation of lack of obtainment—Information that confirms the fact that what is wanted, needed, or expected is not being obtained.
- Confirmation of lack of growth or maturation—Information that confirms the fact that growth or maturation is not being achieved.

### Stages

- Unfreezing—The stage in the change process during which the change agents create dissatisfaction, followed by inspiring the motivation to accept some type of change.
- Moving—A cognitive redefinition by the participants of attitude and behavior toward the planned change.
- Refreezing—The new behaviors are practiced and reinforced.
- Change Agent—The responsible person who moves those to be affected by change through the stages of change in a logical manner.

Curriculum development and change is a complex endeavor that requires nursing education expertise, leadership, and vision. It is a process that should be done often and systematically in order to meet the goals of today's health care systems.

## Planning Learning Within the Curriculum

Planning learning activities requires considerable faculty preparation time. Activities should be planned to enhance critical thinking and can be very important for enhancing students' learning. Planning involves six steps:

- Develop the learning outcomes for the specific learning session
- Creating an anticipatory set
- Selecting a teaching strategy (Refer to Chapter 2 for classroom teaching strategies)
- Considering implementation issues
- Designing closure for the session
- Designing formative and summative evaluation strategies (Jeffries & Norton, 2009, p. 205)

The following sections of this chapter will deal specifically with clinical learning within the curriculum of a nursing program. Clinical learning has long been the hallmark of nursing programs and many of the skills and critical thinking development included in them are dependent on the integration of knowledge within this realm.

## Clinical Teaching and Learning

### The College Learning Laboratory/Resource Center

The college learning laboratory/resource center is the place where students are first introduced to the clinical aspects of the profession. It is a multimedia environment where students use "visual, auditory, kinesthetic, and tactile abilities for the acquisition of cognitive, affective, and psychomotor skills for the lifelong and multidisciplinary learning" (Hodson-Carlton & Worrell-Carlisle, 2009, p. 349). The laboratory may be as simple or as complex as the agency budget allows using the spectrum of low technology or high fidelity technology.

#### Uses of the College Laboratory

- A place for students to learn and practice skills—psychomotor and communication
- A site for competency testing

Planning and cooperation between the classroom teacher and the laboratory instructor is crucial. The content in the laboratory should not conflict or contradict that which is learned in the classroom.

### Simulation

High technology simulation using SIMMAN® and standardized patients is playing a prominent role in the education of nursing students and other health profession students such as physicians, physical and occupational therapists, and psychologists. This technique requires an investment of faculty time, resources, and commitment.

## Definitions

- A simulation resembles reality. In specific reference to health care, simulation is an attempt to "create a safe environment for student learning and to promote standardization of assessment" (Mahara, 1998, p. 1339).
- A simulation is a working representation of reality; it may be an abstracted, simplified, or accelerated model of the process. It allows students to explore systems where the real thing cannot be used for teaching purposes because it involves other people or is too expensive, complex, dangerous, fast, or slow (Gibbs, 1975).
- A simulation is a person, device, or set of conditions that attempts to present evaluation problems authentically. The student or trainee is required to respond to the problems as he or she would under natural circumstances. Frequently, the trainee receives performance feedback as if he or she were in the real situation. Simulation procedures for evaluation and teaching have several common characteristics. The characteristics of simulation are:

  - Trainees see cues and consequences very much like those in the real environment.
  - Trainees can be placed in complex situations.
  - Trainees act as they would in the real environment.
  - The fidelity of a simulation is never completely isomorphic with the "real thing."
  - Simulation can take many forms.
  - Static—as in an anatomical model
  - Automated—using advanced computer technology
  - Some are individual while others are interactive
  - Playful or serious (Scott et al., 2005)

## Evidence-Based Education

Haigh (2007) found that simulation is not just a second best form of learning in the clinical area, but one that offers the potential for deliberation and deep learning. Students have expressed the need for more simulated practice experience. Haigh concluded that there is a need for more well-planned, simulated experiences.

## Selecting Appropriate Clinical Experiences Throughout the Curriculum

Appropriate clinical sites need to be planned throughout the curriculum. They must grow in skill and complexity. The sites must be harmonious with the level outcomes to be achieved and be evaluated frequently to determine if the needs of the student are being met for that curricular level. Clinical experiences must support the outcomes of the program. They must be tied to course objectives and provide practical implementation of the didactic content that has been taught. The clinical instructor must:

- Plan carefully to ensure that students have the opportunity to meet the course objectives.
- Possess knowledge of the content that the students need to master.
- Ensure patient safety.
- Provide opportunity for the students to perform successfully.

The goals of clinical nursing education are to enable the students to:

1. Apply theoretical learning to patient care situations through the use of critical thinking skills to recognize and resolve patient care problems and the use of the nursing process to design therapeutic nursing interventions and evaluate their effectiveness.
2. Develop communication skills in working with patients, their families, and other health care providers.
3. Demonstrate skill in the safe use of therapeutic nursing intervention in providing care to patients
4. Evidence caring behaviors in nursing actions
5. Consider the ethical implication of clinical decision and nursing actions
6. Gain perspective of the contextual environment of health care delivery
7. Experience the various roles of the nurse within the health care delivery system (O'Connor, 2006).

In order to ensure that the above goals are met, Infante (1975) suggested that the essential elements of any clinical experience should include:

- Opportunity for patient contact
- Objectives for activities
- Competent guidance
- Individuation of activities
- Practice for skill learning, both motor and intellectual
- Encouragement of critical thinking
- Opportunity for problem solving
- Opportunity for observation
- Opportunity for experimentation
- Development of professional judgment or decision making
- Encouragement of creative abilities
- Provision for the transfer of knowledge
- Participation in integrative activities
- Utilization of the team concept

## Good Attributes for Clinical Teachers

### Educator Knowledge Attributes

- Knowledge of theory and clinical practice
- Knowledge of the facility
- Knowledge of the student

### Educator Interpersonal Presentation Attributes

- Positive educator attitude
- Encouraging demeanor
- Organizational skill
- Serving as a primary resource

### Teaching Strategies Attributes

- Managing paperwork
- Keeping students challenged
- Post-conference planning (Hanson & Stenvig, 2008)

## Instructional Techniques for the Clinical Setting

One of the goals of the clinical instructor is to assist the student as he or she reflects on their practice (Baker, 1996). A reflective learning practice includes:

- A sense of inner discomfort triggered by a live experience.
- Identification or clarification of the concern makes the nature of the problem or issue more evident.
- Openness to new information from internal and external sources exists, along with the ability to observe and take information from a variety of perspectives; there is a willingness to forego a quick resolution or closure concerning the problem.
- Resolution occurs through insight, where the learner feels she has changed or learned something that is personally significant.
- A change is experienced in self, as a result of internalization of a new perspective.
- A decision is made whether to act on the outcome of their reflective process by determining whether the insight can be operationalized (p. 20).

There is a whole set of strategies available for the clinical teacher that is different from those available to the classroom teacher. Table 5.5 presents selected clinical teaching and supervision strategies, along with some clinical tips for implementing these strategies.

## Evidence-Based Education

Role modeling by nurse educators in the clinical area is closely linked to the perception of competence. Negative role modeling was found to negatively impact students' perceptions of their learning (Charneia, 2007).

| Table 5.5 | Instructional Strategies in the Clinical Area |
|---|---|

**Instructional Strategies**

| Demonstration | The instructor can not only demonstrate physical skills, but also reasoning skills and encourage the student to be attentive to her own mental work. |
|---|---|
| War Stories | War stories describe particularly memorable events in a nurse's past practice that now serve as a paradigm for the students' current practice. |
| Questioning | This is a constant in clinical practice. A form of Socratic questioning will stimulate the students to think the problem through and will elicit formative evaluation. |
| Listening | Clinical faculty must pay careful attention to what the students are saying in the clinical area. Paraphrase the students' comments to ensure clear communication. |

**Supervision of Student Performance of Technical Skills**

| Process of Skill Mastery | Students are at very low levels of skill mastery and will need to go through the sequential steps for all procedures. For information on this process, see Benner (1984). |
|---|---|
| How to Let Go | Faculty need to allow the students to work through their technical skills. Although taking over is a natural skill, do so only if it is absolutely necessary; then allow the student to assume an assistant role. Process the experience with the student. Allow students to ask the patients what works best for them. |
| When to Jump In | The clinical instructor should be prepared to intervene when the student's actions, inaction, or ineptitude jeopardize patient safety. Be calm and assertive. Remember to help the student work through the situation in a way that does not destroy his or her self-esteem. |
| Ensuring that Patient Needs are Met | Help students set priorities so that all care is delivered in a timely manner. Keep the context of the whole situation in mind. The timing of all procedures, as well as the schedule, should be addressed. If the student is caring for more than one patient, help her set priorities. Make sure that the student allows enough time for all activities. |

**Promoting the Integration of Theory and Practice**

| Case Studies | If patients are not available to meet the clinical objectives, preparing case studies that include some of the prescribed objectives will assist the students' learning. |
|---|---|

*(Continued)*

| Table 5.5 | Instructional Strategies in the Clinical Area (Continued) |
|---|---|
| Seminars | Seminars based on patient problems that students have encountered can be used to foster integration. Several students who care for the same patient on different days can work as a group with some of these patients. |
| Nursing Rounds | Nursing rounds involve the whole group. They provide an opportunity for all to reflect on the clinical events. While background information and conclusions are discussed away from the bedside, the patient can add to the discussion by articulating his experience and expectations. |
| Written Assignments | Major nursing care plans, synthesis papers, and journaling may be part of the clinical experiences. Clinical and classroom instructors must collaborate so that students are clear about the assignment. |
| **Developing Critical Thinking Skills and Reflective Practice** | |
| Strategies for Promoting Critical Thinking and Reflective Practice | Clinical instructors must use high order cognitive questioning that includes "why" instead of "what." Debrief all of the experiences in post-conference sessions. Process recordings and self-evaluations to assist the students to think at higher cognitive levels. |

## Making Assignments

Patient assignments should assist the student to tie the course's didactic content to practical applications. Factors to consider are:

- The skill level of the student
- The acuity of the patient
- The number of students in the clinical group
- The availability of patients whose conditions directly meet the objectives of the day

Types of assignments can also differ in order to meet the clinical objectives and include:

- *Dual Assignments:* Should be used when the complexity of care is more than one student can handle. The faculty is responsible for making sure each student is clear about his or her role in this situation.
- *Observational Assignments:* Should be used to augment the student's appreciation of the various procedures that patients experience but where there is not a reason for them to practice. Faculty can send students to the operating room, radiology or lab departments, clinics, etc to observe.

Considerations for making clinical assignments are listed here (O'Connor, 2006).

1. Assess available clinical material

   ▪ What experiences are available in the clinical setting?

   ▪ What potential learning opportunities are presented in relation to specialty-specific theoretical content, skill development, overriding curricular content (e.g., interpersonal communication, patient teaching, advocacy, life span development, etc.)?

   ▪ What anticipated patient events (e.g., absence from the unit for prolonged testing, imminent discharge) might interrupt or interfere with student learning?

   ▪ Have staff voiced concerns or cautions regarding specific patient care assignments?

2. What are the curricular goals and related clinical objectives for this experience?

   ▪ What is the primary focus of learning for this clinical experience?

   ▪ Can that focus be described as a larger concept of which the specific patient case at hand is an example?

   ▪ What other learning can be extracted from the situation? Scan curricular goals and clinical objectives to identify two or three other objectives that might be addressed in the experience.

   ▪ Does the student have sufficient background knowledge, either from previous courses or experiences or from the concurrent theoretical class, to deal with the situation? If not, can sufficient theory be provided to permit the student to function safely and effectively in an otherwise excellent learning situation?

3. What is the overall environment for learning?

   ▪ Can connections be made between the proposed assignment and the previous experiences of the student that will help to integrate the experiences?

   ▪ What lessons might be drawn from the specific clinical setting that can be carried over into another setting (e.g., what information from the patient setting would be helpful to the nurse providing care for the patient in a community setting or to the nurse providing care for a nursing home resident admitted to the hospital for an episodic illness)?

   ▪ What staffing issues need to be considered in making the assignment (e.g., short staffing because of illness or planned meetings) that may impact the learning experience?

4. What do you, as the instructor, feel comfortable managing?

   ▪ Where do you anticipate needing to spend the most time with specific students and/or specific patient care assignments?

   ▪ Does the overall assignment shortchange any students or create safety issues?

   ▪ What patient events can or might happen in the course of the clinical day? If one or more of these events were to occur, would this be manageable given the assignments planned for all students in the group?

5. What are the characteristics of the learner group and individual students?

- What previous experiences have the students had that can be drawn on when managing the proposed clinical assignment?
- What is the performance level of individual students? Is each student capable of managing the proposed assignment?
- Has each student had opportunities to progress toward achieving clinical objectives?
- What level of independent functioning has each student achieved? Will one or more students require more attention than others?
- What learning needs have individual students expressed? Are these addressed in the assignment?
- Have students voiced any specific needs or desires in relation to clinical assignments? Can these be accommodated?
- What is the level of student confidence? Anxiety?
- Can each student function safely? If not, what precautions must be taken as the student proceeds through the clinical day?
- Are there any special needs of patients that can be matched to a student's special abilities?

6. What backup plans are available?

- Can students be paired in providing care without diluting the experience?
- Can students be assigned multiple patients to provide opportunities to practice planning and priority setting when challenging clinical situations are not available?
- Are there any off-unit experiences available that address clinical objectives?
- Can students focus on a single skill set with multiple patients?
- Can case studies and "what if" scenarios be developed to use "down time" effectively?

## Pre- and Postconference

The clinical day requires thought and preparation in order for the students to successfully apply the knowledge that they have learned in the classroom to patient care. The preconference is a time to review the clinical objectives, the kinds of patients the students will care for, the degree of preparation the students have done, and any procedures that may be part of the day. Whether this is done in a formal setting with all students present, or done informally and individually with each student, will depend on the level of the student and the instructor's preference. The goal is to be sure that all students are adequately prepared. Postconference is a time for students to process the day's experiences. O'Conner (2006) discussed the purposes of the session.

- Providing a time for both student and instructor to pause and reflect on the day's events, their meaning, and the relation between what has been observed and experienced and what was taught in the classroom or discussed in assigned readings.

- Contributing to the achievement of course and clinical objectives by making explicit the connections between clinical activities and the goals for learning.
- Examining commonalities and differences in patient responses to illness and its treatment within the clinical specialty.
- Permitting students to vicariously share in their peers' experiences, broadening their exposure to the clinical situations they might encounter in practice.
- Promoting affective learning through debriefing that allows students to express feelings and attitudes about the experiences they encountered during the day's activities.
- Providing students with experience in the effective use of the group process.

## The Affective Domain in Clinical Practice

The AACN (1998) identified five core values that epitomize the caring, professional nurse.

- *Altruism* is a concern for the welfare and well being of others. In professional practice, altruism is reflected by the nurse's concern and advocacy for the welfare of patients, other nurses, and other health care providers.
- *Autonomy* is the right of self-determination. Professional practice reflects autonomy when the nurse respects patients' rights to make decisions about their health care.
- *Human Dignity* is respect for the inherent worth and uniqueness of individuals and populations. In professional practice, concern for human dignity is reflected when the nurse values and respects all patients and colleagues.
- *Integrity* is acting in accordance with an appropriate code of ethics and accepted standards of practice. Integrity is reflected in professional practice when the nurse is honest and provides care based on an ethical framework that is accepted within the profession.
- *Social Justice* is acting in accordance with fair treatment regardless of economic status, ethnicity, age, citizenship, disability, or sexual orientation.

These core values come into play in the clinical area where the clinical instructor must be alert to demonstrate how these values inform patient care. Opportunities are present in every clinical experience to apply ethical principles, but often students need to be prompted to examine their performance and attitudes in light of these values.

## Strategies for Evaluating Student Learning in the Clinical Area

While evaluation of student performance in the clinical area is vital, the faculty member needs to remember that teaching is primary. Students need clear definitions of safe and unsafe behavior, and faculty need to give very specific rationales for their decision to give an unsatisfactory grade. On the other hand, the teacher should remember that often the first time a student performs a procedure, he or she may need some coaching. There is a fine line between teaching and evaluating in the clinical area. Table 5.6 presents a variety of evaluation methods that are useful when evaluating students' clinical performance. They include:

- Observation of students as they perform in the clinical area
- Student written work that is used to reveal intellectual processes that guide students' clinical performance
- Oral presentations
- Simulations
- Student self-evaluation
- Testimonials from staff

Frequent feedback (daily if possible) is essential for students to have the opportunity to improve on areas found to be deficient. Without positive and frequent feedback, the goal of the clinical experience can be lost.

# CASE STUDY

## Case Study 5.1

*Dr. Linda Wilson and Dr. Fran Cornelius contributed this case study.*
Marjorie is a seasoned nursing faculty member at a major university. She has been asked by the Dean to serve as the curriculum coordinator and a mentor to a new faculty member, Stephanie. Stephanie is also on the curriculum committee and comes to the university with 8 years' teaching experience at a mid-sized university. Discuss the mentor-mentee relationship in this situation. What are some of the assets Marjorie and Stephanie can bring to the curriculum committee? How should Marjorie approach this responsibility? What are the key elements of mentorship that she should be certain to address? What is Stephanie's responsibility in this relationship?

## Practice Questions

1. Planning for curriculum development should include which activity?
   A. Analyzing the beliefs of the faculty teaching support courses
   B. Collecting the demographic data of the community
   C. Diagnosing the faculty's learning styles
   D. Advising the parent institution's president that the curriculum will change

| Table 5.6 | Clinical Evaluation Methods |
|---|---|

**Observation**—Observations of students as they perform in the clinical area

| | |
|---|---|
| Anecdotal Notes | The means by which data is obtained through observation and recorded for later evaluation |
| Incident Reports | Instances of unsafe behavior. If no other instances of unsafe behavior occur, the event should be ignored in the student's final evaluation. |
| Rating Scales | Provide a summary of accumulated observations of the student's clinical performance. These scales are usually based on the course objectives. |
| External Raters | A rating done by a person who has not seen the student perform previously. |
| Videotapes | Videotapes can be recorded in a simulated setting. They are also of value in distance learning settings. |
| Skills Checklist | Skills checklists are usually used in the college laboratory and detail the steps for a particular skill. They can be used for teaching as well as learning. |

**Written Work**—reveals the intellectual processes that guide students' clinical performances

| | |
|---|---|
| Observation Guides | These guides can be developed to assist the students in observing an independent assignment or off-unit experience |
| Process Recordings | Process recordings are used to capture interpersonal interactions between the student and another person. They focus on communication skills. |
| Nursing Care Plans | The major nursing care plan details the application of the nursing process for all nursing diagnoses that the student has identified for a selected patient. |

*Oral Presentations*—Includes communication with staff and instructors, active participation in pre and post conference, and formal presentations.

*Simulations*—May also be used for evaluation and teaching. This standardizes the stimuli to which students respond. Simulations may be in the form of a case study, the use of manikins or models, or standardized patients.

*Self-Evaluation*—Often students provide valuable insights for their instructors when they conduct a self-evaluation.

*Testimonial*—Verbal comments from staff, patients and, in some cases, other students may play a part in the evaluation process. However, the instructor should validate the observation herself.

Adapted from *Clinical Instruction and Evaluation: A Resource Guide* (2nd ed.), by A. O'Connor, 2006, Chapter 9. Sudbury, MA: Jones and Bartlett Publishers; and "Strategies for Evaluating Learning Outcomes," by J. M. Kilpatrick, D. DeWittt-Weaver, & L. Yeager, 2009, Chapter 21. In D. M. Billings & J. A. Halstead (Eds.), *Teaching in Nursing: A Guide for Faculty*. St. Louis, MO: Elsevier.

2. When choosing a leader for a curriculum revision, the faculty should consider which of the following first?
   A. The specific work involved
   B. The personality of the leader
   C. The skill level of the learners
   D. The creativity of the committee members

3. A faculty member insists that her favorite disease, juvenile thrombocytopenic purpera, be included in the pediatric syllabus despite her colleagues' concerns. Which is the best strategy for the leader to take?
   A. Demand that she remove the content from her syllabus
   B. Advise her to publish an article about the disease
   C. Remind her of her responsibility to adhere to the curriculum plan
   D. Counsel her to become a clinical specialist in a pediatric hospital

4. When developing the curriculum, the faculty will look to which of the following for their reason of being?
   A. Professional standards and guidelines
   B. Nursing theory and research
   C. Institutional mission/philosophy
   D. Community and societal needs

5. A graduate of the program identifies nursing as assessing, planning, implementing, and evaluating the care of clients and families with various health care needs. He most likely comes from a program model that is known as
   A. Curriculum model
   B. Integrated model
   C. Nursing theorist model
   D. Deconstructed model

6. Which curriculum model would include a course titled "Nursing Care of Clients with Respiratory Problems Across the Life Span"?
   A. Curriculum model
   B. Integrated model
   C. Nursing theorist model
   D. Deconstructed model

7. When considering level outcomes, the educator must ensure that they progress logically to eventually reflect the:
   A. Philosophy of the parent institution
   B. Outcomes of the program
   C. Demographics of the community
   D. Beliefs of the faculty

8. A nurse should use which of the following teaching strategies to reach the higher levels of Bloom's Taxonomy?
   A. Lecture
   B. Discussion
   C. Demonstration
   D. Questioning

9. The students in your clinical group have requested that you provide them with some additional materials that will help them study for their next examination. What independent strategy would be appropriate?
   A. Extra journal articles to read
   B. A tape of your lecture
   C. A game addressing the material
   D. Some role-playing scenarios

10. Which teaching strategy requires considerable student preparation?
    A. Collaborative learning
    B. Simulation
    C. Debate
    D. Role play

## References

American Association of Colleges of Nursing (AACN). (2008). *The essentials of baccalaureate education for professional nursing practice.* Washington, DC: Author.

American Association of University Professors. (1940, 1970). Statement of principles on academic freedom and tenure with interpretive comments. Retrieved October 13, 2008, from http://www.aaup.org/statement/Redbook/1940

The American Heritage Dictionary of the English Language. (1970). Third Edition. Boston, MA: Houghton Mifflin Company.

Baker, C. (1996). Clinical education: A teaching strategy for critical thinking. *Journal of Nursing Education, 35,* 19–22.

Barnum, B. J. (1998). The advanced nurse practitioner: Struggling toward a conceptual framework. *Nursing Leadership Forum, 3*(1), 14–17.

Benner, P. (1984). From novice to expert: excellence and power in clinical nursing practice. Reading, MA: Addison-Wesley Publishing.

Charneia, E. (2007). *Nursing students' perceptions of role modeling as it relates to learning in the clinical environment.* Unpublished manuscript. Capella University.

Finke, L. M. (2009). Teaching in nursing: The faculty role. In D. M. Billings & J. A. Halstead (Eds.), *Teaching in nursing: a guide for faculty.* St. Louis, MO: Elsevier.

Gibbs, G. C. (1975). *Academic gaming and simulation in education and training: Proceedings of a conference jointly organised by the Society for Academic Gaming and Simulation.* London: Kogan.

Goad, S., & Hough, L. (1993). Lewin's field theory with emphasis on change. In S. Zeigler (Ed.), *Theory-directed nursing practice* (pp. 183–192). New York: Springer Publishing.

Haigh, J. (2007). Expansive learning in the university setting: The case for simulated clinical experiences. *Nurse Education in Practice, 7,* 95–102.

Halstead, J. A., Rains, J., Boland, D. L., & May, R. (1996). Reconceptualizing baccalaureate nursing education: Outcomes and competencies for practice in the 21st century. *Journal of Nursing Education, 35*(9), 413–416.

Hanson, K., & Stenvig, T. E. (2008). The good clinical nursing educator and the baccalaureate nursing clinical experience: Attributes and praxis. *Journal of Nursing Education, 47*(1), 38–42.

Hodson-Carlton, K. E., & Worrell-Carlisle, P. J. (2009). The learning resource center. In D. M. Billings & J. A. Halstead (Eds.), *Teaching in nursing: A guide for faculty.* St. Louis, MO: Elsevier.

Huber, D. (2000). *Leadership and nursing care management* (2nd ed.). Philadelphia: W.B. Saunders.

Infante, M. S. (1975). *The clinical laboratory in nursing education.* New York: John Wiley & Sons, Inc.

Ironsides, P. (2004). "Covering content" and teaching thinking: Deconstructing the additive curriculum. *Journal of Nursing Education, 43*(1), 5–12.

Jeffries, P., & Norton, B. (2009). Selecting learning activities to achieve curriculum outcomes. In D. M. Billings & J. A. Halstead (Eds.), *Teaching in nursing: A guide for faculty* (pp. 205–212). St. Louis, MO: Elsevier

Keating, S. (2006). *Curriculum development and evaluation in nursing.* Philadelphia: Lippincott Williams & Wilkins.

Kilpatrick, J. M., DeWittt-Weaver, D., & Yeager, L. (2009). Strategies for evaluating learning outcomes. In D. M. Billings & J. A. Halstead (Eds.), *Teaching in nursing: A guide for faculty.* St. Louis, MO: Elsevier.

Leddy, S. (2007). Curriculum development in Nursing Education. In B. Moyer & R. A. Wittmann-Price (Eds.), *Foundations of Practice Excellence* (pp. 66–81). Philadelphia: F.A. Davis Company.

Mahara, M. (1998). A perspective on clinical evaluation in nursing education. *Journal of Advanced Nursing, 28,* 1339–1346.

McDonald, M. (2007). *The nurse educator's guide to assessing learning outcomes.* Sudbury, MA: Jones and Bartlett Publishers.

Mind Tools. (n.d.). Retrieved April 2, 2009, from http://www.mindtools.com/pages/artoc;e/newLDC_84.htm

Morris, W. (Ed.). (1970). *The American heritage dictionary of the English language.* Boston: American Heritage Publishing Co., Inc and Houghton Mifflin Company.

National League for Nursing. (1993). *A vision for nursing education.* New York: Author.

National League for Nursing. (2005). Core competencies of nurse educators with task statements. Retrieved May 1, 2009, from www.nln.org

National League for Nursing Accrediting Commission (NLNAC). (2008). *Standards and criteria.* Retrieved April 3, 3009, from: http://www.nlnac.com/manuals/SC2008.htm

O'Connor, A. (2006). *Clinical instruction and evaluation: A resource guide* (2nd ed.). Sudbury, MA: Jones and Bartlett Publishers.

Scott, J. A., Issenberg, S. B., Miller, G. T., & Brotons, A. A. (2005). Fake it: how to create a simulation training program. *Homeland First Response, 3*(3), 12–17.

Team Technology. (2008). Retrieved April 2, 2009, from http://www.teamtechnology.co.uk/

Walker, D., & Soltis, J. (2004). *Curriculum and aims.* New York: Teachers College Press.

Webber, P. B. (2002). A curriculum framework for nursing. *Journal of Nursing Education, 41*(1), 1524.

Wiles, J., & Bondi, J. (1998). *Curriculum development: A guide to practice* (5th ed.). Upper Saddle River, NJ: W. B. Saunders Canada.

Wirth, R. (2004). Lewin/Schein's Change Theory. Retrieved on May 16, 2009, from http://www.entarga.com/orgchange/lewinschein.pdf

Yoder-Wise, P. (1995). *Loading and managing in nursing.* St. Louis, MO: Mosby Year Book.

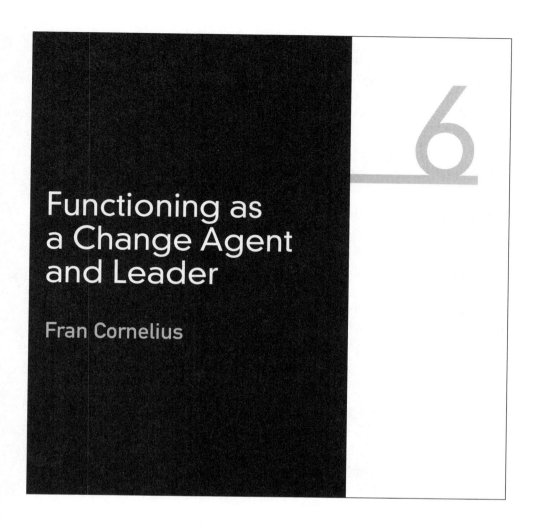

# Functioning as a Change Agent and Leader

Fran Cornelius

*Education is not preparation for life; education is life itself.*

—John Dewey

**NLN Core Competency V: Function as a Change Agent and Leader**

Nurse educators function as change agents and leaders to create a preferred future for nursing education and nursing practice (National League for Nursing [NLN], 2005, p. 20).

**Learning Outcomes**

- Discuss the importance of cultural sensitivity when advocating for change.
- Discuss the effect of organizational culture on the climate of innovation within nursing education.
- Identify strategies to support a climate of creativity and innovation within nursing education.
- Identify measures to evaluate organizational effectiveness in nursing education.

■ Analyze the nurse educator's leadership role with respect to creating an environment of innovation.

■ Analyze strategies that drive organizational change.

■ Elaborate on strategies for integrating a long-term, innovative, and creative perspective into the nurse educator role.

■ Elaborate on the importance of collaboration with the larger academic community to expand the learning environment.

## Introduction

This chapter will focus on the nurse educator's role as a leader who interfaces with the larger academic community and administration, the role of the nurse educator within the larger system, and becoming a change agent within a variety of systems.

## The Nurse Educator's Role as a Leader and Change Agent

### Overview

Mahoney (2001) states the essential qualities of a nurse leader include: having competence, confidence, courage, creativity, collaboration, and therapeutic communication skills. In addition:

> Nursing administrators, educators and clinicians have a responsibility to keep abreast of health care's rapidly changing environment and make changes proactively. In order for nurses to create change they must be aware of the key issues effecting the nursing profession. (p. 271)

> Opportunities abound for nurses to lead, but few are born leaders: Most must learn effective leadership skills. Paying attention to and developing four simple things—having followers, moving in the right direction, setting examples, and having authenticity—enable nurses to be effective leaders. The challenge lies in continually acting and questioning what can be done to make a difference. (Dickenson-Hazard, 2004, p. 145)

The functions of a nurse leader include:

1. "Acting as a role model for others
2. Providing expert nursing care based on theory and research findings
3. Demonstrating knowledge about organizational theory to support and influence organizational policies
4. Collaborating with others to provide optimum health care
5. Assuming responsibility for providing information and support to patients
6. Using advocacy to help effect changes that will benefit patients and the health care organization
7. Using the nursing codes of ethics and standards of practice as guidelines for individual and professional accountability" (Grant & Massey, 1999, as cited in Mahoney, 2001 p. 270)

## Skills and Attributes of a Leader

Carroll (2005) conducted a study to compare the perceptions of female leaders and nurse executives about what skills and attributes would be needed to succeed in the 21st century. Six factors were identified:

1. *Personal integrity:* includes adherence to ethical standards, trustworthiness, and credibility.
2. *Strategic vision/action orientation:* related to creating and articulating a vision of a preferred future, managing change, seeing possibilities instead of obstacles, exhibiting a determination to succeed and a commitment to action, being proactive, evaluating, being resilient, promoting excellence, and seeing the big picture. (p. 149)
3. *Team building/communication:* skills to build coalitions, make effective oral presentations, debate and discuss important issues, build a team, and build consensus.
4. *Management and technical competence:* "ability to make decisions, think critically, solve problems, plan, direct, organize, control, and be technically competent in a field, profession or discipline" (p. 150).
5. *People skills:* ability to empower others, network, value diversity, and work collaboratively.
6. *Personal survival skills/attributes:* political sensitivity, self-direction, self-reliance, courage, a competitive and entrepreneurial spirit, and candor.

## Competencies Associated With Leadership

Longest (1998) identified six critical leadership competencies in health care today. These include:

1. *Conceptual:* Knowledge and skill to envision one's place in the organization within larger society.
2. *Technical:* Direct work performed in one's domain.
3. *Interpersonal or collaborative:* Human interactions and relations through which one leads others in pursuit of common objectives.
4. *Political:* Dual capacity to accurately assess the impact of public policies on the performance of one's domain of responsibility and the ability to influence public policymaking at both state and federal levels.
5. *Commercial:* Economic exchanges between buyers and sellers in which value is created.
6. *Governance:* Establishment and enactment of a clear vision for the organization.

Green (2006) also identifies several critical competencies for nurse educators that relate to the role of a change agent and leader. These include:

- Collaboration
  - Teamwork: An essential component of the nurse educator's role
  - Developing networks and partnerships to improve nursing's influence within the community

## Evidence-Based Education

> Competent leadership skills are needed to manage today's chaotic health care environment. Lack of leadership competence contributes to employee frustration and dissatisfaction, which directly and indirectly impacts the supply of health care workers. To address this problem, the Arizona nursing community designed a Leadership Model based on six critical leadership competencies needed in today's health care environment. This has become a 4-day educational program offering. They report 100% participant completion rates (Weston et al., 2008).
>
> Using a Robert Wood Johnson Colleague in Caring grant, The Arizona Health Care Leadership Academy developed and now provides a successful model for creating a statewide partnership for providing a high-quality, cost-effective, locally offered leadership education program (Weston et al., 2008).

- Working with faculty and students to support progress toward the achievement of realistic and optimal learning goals.
- Conferring with nursing leadership to make recommendations and develop educational interventions.

- Systems Thinking

  - "Involves the ability of the nurse educator to incorporate the body of knowledge, resources, and tools available within and outside the healthcare system to optimize learning experiences and teaching opportunities" (p. 279).
  - Focuses on interrelationships and how these impact the process of change and are, in turn, affected by this process.
  - Identifying the social, economic, political, and institutional forces influencing nursing education.

- Advocacy/Moral Agency

  - Monitor legal and ethical issues relevant to higher education and nursing education, and act to influence, plan, and implement policies and procedures.
  - Decisions and actions guided by ethical principles grounded in an appreciation of cultural diversity and individual rights.

Nelson, Godfrey, and Purdy (2004) studied hospital mentoring programs. They found that hospitals that used a mentorship program spent less and realized great benefits. It was a successful way to recruit and retain the brightest graduate nurses. Hospital-based mentorship programs increase recruitment and retention and are cost effective (Nelson et al., 2004). Mentors are nurses who facilitate learning and emulate leadership skills.

There are three theoretical perspectives that explain how a person can become a leader:

- *Trait Theory:* A "natural-born" leader possesses natural leadership traits that lead him or her into leadership roles.

- *Great Events Theory:* An ordinary person responds to a crisis or disastrous event and emerges as a leader.
- *Transformational Leadership:* A person chooses to become a leader by seeking opportunities to develop leadership skills (Bass, 1990; Clark, 2008).

In order to develop leadership skills, a nurse educator must assume the responsibility of seeking out opportunities for professional development. It is essential to take the initiative to obtain an accurate assessment of one's current leadership skills and performance.

- This process can be started by creating a list of strengths and weaknesses.
- Typically, it is fairly easy to identify strengths, but most people find it difficult to identify weaknesses.
- The nurse educator must seek out opportunities to develop leadership skills, link with potential leadership mentors and coaches, and actively solicit very specific feedback from a variety of sources.
- It is essential to be receptive to feedback and reflect on it throughout the process.

## Essential Leadership Skills

Sarros, Cooper, and Santora (2008) found that "transformational leadership is linked with organizational culture primarily through the process of articulating vision, and, to a lesser extent, through setting of high-performance expectations and providing individual support" (p. 155). Leadership and organizational culture are widely believed to be linked in the process of change.

*Sources of Influence.* Creative and innovative leaders must embody the following traits and abilities:

- "Organizational understanding" and political skills
- Creative thinking skills for idea evaluation
- Self-awareness
- Adaptability in changing environments and, as deficiencies emerge, be able to adapt further through "the utilization of compensatory strategies" (Mumford, Connelly, & Gaddis, 2003).
- Collaborative thinking. Creative work frequently involves collaboration with other disciplines, as well as with non-traditional partners. Looking for partnerships outside one's usual circles can lead to successful, win-win partnerships (Glasgow & Cornelius, 2005).
- Integration-minded. Leaders are more effective when using an integrative style that permits him or her to orchestrate expertise, people, and relationships in such a way as to bring new ideas into being. There are three critical elements to this integrative style of leadership:
  - *Idea generation:* Stresses the role of the leader in facilitating others' idea generation
  - *Idea structuring:* Refers to guidance with respect to the technical and organizational merits of the work, setting output expectations, and identifying and integrating the projects to be pursued

- *Idea promotion:* "Involves gathering support form the broader organization for the creative enterprise as a whole as well as implementation of a specific idea or project" (Mumford, Scott, Gaddis, & Strange, 2002, pp. 738–739)

In other words, making sure the resources (time, staff, funds, etc.) to complete the project are available.

## Evaluating Organizational Effectiveness

Research has called for organizations to be more flexible, adaptive, entrepreneurial, and innovative to meet the changing demands of today's environment more effectively (Sarros, Cooper, & Santora, 2008). Additional research has found that organizational performance is linked to participative leadership and an innovative organizational culture (Ogbonna & Harris, 2000).

Thibodeaux and Favilla (1996) define organizational effectiveness as the "extent to which an organization, by the use of certain resources, fulfils its objectives without depleting its resources and without placing undue strain on its members and/or society" (p. 21). There are a number of models that facilitate the evaluation of organizational effectiveness. Many of the models of organizational effectiveness have similar attributes, and include:

- Clear goals that are well communicated
- Resources allocated to innovation and change
- Members (faculty) are satisfied
- There is marketing of the success
- Education is rewarded
- Planning for the future (Cheng, 1996)

Scott (1996) states that, "in order to evaluate effectiveness, it is necessary first to establish standards to use for comparison to actual performance. Specific evaluation criteria are based on outcomes, on processes, and on structures" (p. 353).

## Outcomes

- "Focus is on materials or objects on which the organization has performed some operation" (Scott, 1996, p. 353)
- Are the most common effectiveness measurement
- Are difficult to define and measure, therefore a frequent problem is ambiguity and measurement error

## Processes

- "Assess effort rather than effect" (Scott, 1996, p. 355)
- Measure work quantity or quality
- Substituting process criteria for outcome criteria can compromise service

## Structures

- "Structural indicators assess the capacity of the organization for effective performance" (Scott, 1996, p. 357)
- Indicators include:

  - Organizational features (equipment age or type)
  - Participant characteristics (degree attained, licensing, etc.)

- Form the basis for accreditation reviews and licensing systems (Scott, 1996).

## Establishing a Culture of Change

An organization's climate and culture have a significant impact upon creativity and innovation displayed within it.

- Climate is defined as "people's perceptions of organizational interactions and characteristics" (Mumford et al., 2002, p. 732).
- Culture is defined as the "normative expectations for desirable behavior" which determines, to a large extent, how people act within that organization (Mumford et al., 2002, p. 732).
- The predominant view is that organizational culture cannot be "managed," however "certain contingencies (such as crises or leadership turnover) may present the opportunity to *influence* organizational culture" (Martin & Meyerson, 1988, p. 783).

While a source of influence may be a crisis or leadership change, there are other sources of influence that can drive change. Grenny et al. (2008) state that effective change agents "drive change by relying on several different sources of influence strategies at the same time. . . .

- By combining multiple sources of influence, they are up to 10 times more successful at producing substantial and sustainable change" (p. 47).
- Grenny also identifies six sources of influences that a nurse educator can utilize to influence change. Those sources are divided into motivation and ability under the realms of personal, social, and structural influences. An example of personal motivation to change occurs when the change is valued and the ability for personal change comes with education. Social motivation to change may come in the form of peer pressure but the social ability to change uses a supportive environment. Structural motivators to change may come in the form of incentives and the ability is found in organizational structures that support change. Nurse educators can effect change if they reflect on the motivational and ability aspects of change within the personal, social, and structural systems in which they function.

Many studies have identified interactional factors that foster an environment of creativity and innovation (Mumford, Connelly, & Gaddis, 2003). These factors include:

1. Risk taking
2. Freedom
3. Work challenge
4. Openness
5. Trust
6. Support
7. Intellectual orientation
8. Intrinsic involvement
9. Activity/experimentation

The presence of these interacting factors influences the individual's perception of the organization's openness to creativity, and consequently affects (Ekvall & Ryhammer, 1999):

- His/her willingness to initiate creative efforts
- The rate of idea generation
- The likely success of implementation efforts

## The Process of Change

Nauheimer (2005) states that sustained change requires transformation on three levels: individual, team/unit, and organization or larger system. Successful change can be better understood and facilitated through the lens of a change theory.

- In this process, the nurse educator can assist in the identification of positive opportunities for change and strategies to effectively manage change, whether planned or unplanned.
- The nurse leader must not only have skill in applying change theory, but also have a keen understanding of what interventions will affect, encourage, and manage the change process.
- It is essential to keep in mind that not all change is improvement, but all improvement is change (White, 2004).

## The Nurse Leader as a Change Agent

Acquiring and incorporating the skill sets of effective change agents can help nurse leaders to implement any change successfully. These skills include the ability to:

- Combine ideas from unconnected sources
- Energize others by keeping the interest level up and demonstrating a high personal energy level

- Develop skill in human relations, such as well-developed interpersonal communication skills, group management, and problem-solving skills
- Retain a big-picture focus while dealing with each part of the system
- Be flexible and willing to modify ideas if the modification will improve the change, but to resist nonproductive tampering with the implementation
- Be confident and avoid the tendency to be easily discouraged
- Think realistically regarding how quickly staff will accept and perform new processes competently
- Be trustworthy, with a track record of integrity and success through other systemic changes
- Articulate a vision through insights and versatile thinking to instill confidence in others
- Be able to handle resistance to a new process (White, 2004).

## Change Theories

The predominant models of change include:

1. Lewin's Three-Step Change Theory
2. Lippitt's Phases of Change Theory
3. Prochaska and DiClemente's Change Theory
4. Social Cognitive Theory
5. Theory of Reasoned Action
6. Theory of Planned Behavior

## Characteristics of Various Change Models

### Lewin's Three-Step Change Theory

Lewin's Three-Step Change Theory sees change as a dynamic balance of forces working in opposing directions.

- Driving forces:

  - Facilitate change
  - Push individuals/organizations in the desired direction for change

- Restraining forces:

  - Hinder change
  - Push individuals/organizations in the opposite direction of the desired change
  - Forces must be analyzed and manipulated to shift the balance in the direction of the planned change

- Lewin's model is very rational and goal- and plan-oriented
- It does not take into account personal factors that can affect change

### Lippitt's Phases of Change Theory

- Lippitt's Phases of Change Theory is an extension of Lewin's Three-Step Theory, and focuses on the *change agent,* rather than the change itself.
- Lippitt's theory includes seven steps:
  1. Diagnose the problem.
  2. Assess the motivation and capacity for change.
  3. Assess the resources and motivation of the change agent. This includes the change agent's commitment to change, power, and stamina.
  4. Choose progressive change objects. In this step, action plans are developed and strategies are established.
  5. The role of the change agents should be selected and clearly understood by all parties so that expectations are clear. Examples of roles are: cheerleader, facilitator, and expert.
  6. Maintain the change. Communication, feedback, and group coordination are essential elements in this step of the change process.
  7. Gradually terminate from the helping relationship. "The change agent should gradually withdraw from their role over time. This will occur when the change becomes part of the organizational culture" (Lippitt, Watson, & Westley, pp. 58–59, as cited by Kritsonis, 2004–2005).

### Prochaska and DiClemente's Change Theory

Prochaska and DiClemente's Change Theory considers change from the perspective that a person moves through stages of change. The stages are:

1. Precontemplation
2. Contemplation
3. Preparation
4. Action
5. Maintenance

- Prochaska and DiClemente's model is cyclical, not linear.
- It takes relapses or failures into account. Individuals who relapse can revisit the contemplation stage and make plans for action in the future (Kritsonis, 2004–2005).

### Social Cognitive Theory (Social Learning Theory)

- In Social Cognitive Theory, self-efficacy is the most important characteristic and must be present for successful change. "Self-efficacy is defined as having the confidence in the ability to take action and persist in the action" (Kritsonis, 2004–2005, p. 6).
- Social Cognitive Theory proposes that behavioral change is affected by environmental influences and personal factors.
- This theory takes into account both external and internal environmental conditions (Grizzell, 2007; Kritsonis, 2004–2005).

### Theory of Reasoned Action

- Theory of Reasoned Action states that a person's actions are determined by his or her intention to perform that action.
- Intention is determined by two major factors:
  - The person's attitude toward the behavior or change (i.e., beliefs about the outcomes of the behavior and the value of these outcomes).
  - The influence of the person's social environment or subjective norms (i.e., beliefs about what other people think the person should do, as well as the person's motivation to comply with the opinions of others (Grizzell, 2007; Kritsonis, 2004–2005).

### Theory of Planned Behavior

- The Theory of Planned Behavior expands upon the Theory of Reasoned Action by including the concept of the individual's perceived control over the opportunities, resources, and skills necessary to perform a behavior or change. This perception of control is believed to be a critical facet of behavior change processes (Grizzell, 2007).
- As with the Social Cognitive Theory, self-efficacy is an important characteristic and must be present for successful change.

### Diffusion of Innovation Theory

Rogers's Diffusion of Innovation Theory provides insight into the process by which new ideas are disseminated and integrated. It can be both spontaneous and planned. "The main elements in the diffusion are:

1. An innovation
2. That is *communicated* through certain *channels*
3. *Over time*
4. Among the members of a *social system.*" (Rogers, 2003, p. 35)

In order for diffusion to be successful, it is absolutely essential to have key people and policy makers interested in the innovation and committed to its implementation. This theory further identifies the five steps in the process of innovation diffusion as:

1. *Knowledge:* The decision-making unit is introduced to the innovation and begins to understand it.
2. *Persuasion:* An attitude, favorable or unfavorable, forms toward the innovation.
3. *Decision:* Activities lead to a decision to adopt or reject the innovation.
4. *Implementation:* The innovation is put to use, and reinvention or alterations may occur.
5. *Confirmation:* "The individual or decision-making unit seeks reinforcement that the decision was correct. If there are conflicting messages or experiences, the original decision may be reversed" (White, 2004, pp. 50–51).

Rogers (2003) describes diffusion as a "kind of *social change,* defined as the process by which alteration occurs in the structure and function of a social system. When new ideas are invented, diffused, and adopted or rejected, leading to certain consequences, social change occurs" (p. 6). Berwick (2003) uses Rogers's theory to explain the rate of change and states that the rate correlates to the following:

1. Perceptions of the innovation/change

   ■ Perceived benefit of the change
   ■ Compatibility with the values, beliefs, past history, and current needs of individuals
   ■ Level of complexity of the proposed innovation or change. The rate of change for simpler changes is generally faster than those that are more complex
   ■ "Re-invention" of the innovation or change (the adaptability of the change). The capability of making local (or point of use) modifications, which often involves simplification, is a common characteristic of successful dissemination
   ■ Changes spread faster when they have these five perceived attributes: benefit, compatibility, simplicity, trialability (ability to "test the waters"), and observability.

2. Characteristics of the people who either adopt the innovation or do not:

   ■ The curve of adoption of the innovation or change over time is generally an S-shape, characterized with an early slow phase affecting a very few individuals (early adopters), a rapid middle phase with widespread adoption, followed by a slow third phase, typically ending with incomplete adoption. It has been described as being similar to the epidemic curve of a contagious disease.
   ■ Rogers's (2003) Diffusion of Innovations Theory includes five levels of adoption. (For more information, see Figure 6.1.)

## 6.1   Rogers's adopter categories.

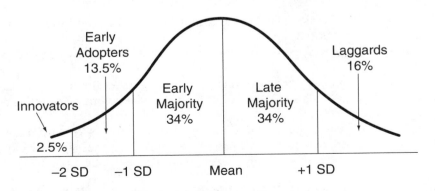

Time to Adoption (SDs From Mean)

- Innovators
- Early Adopters
- Early Majority
- Late Majority
- Laggards

Contextual factors: These include situational/environmental factors associated with a particular organization or social system such as management, leadership, communication or incentives that can either "encourage and support, or discourage and impede, the actual processes" of diffusion (Berwick, 2003, p. 1972).

## Cultural Sensitivity When Advocating for Change

Individuals' ethnic identities and cultural backgrounds strongly influence their attitudes, values, and practices. When advocating for change, it is essential that the nurse educator consider these qualities and act in a culturally sensitive manner. The attributes Meleis (1999) identified that can be integrated into the change process include:

- Culturally competent care is care that is sensitive to the differences individuals may have in their experiences and responses due to their heritage, sexual orientation, socioeconomic situation, ethnicity, and cultural background.
- "A culturally competent person is a person who is able to recognize differences, identify similar patterns of responses, avoid stereotyping by acknowledging variations, and balance his or her own caring actions" (p. 12).

The essential cultural competencies relevant to the process of advocating for change include:

- Awareness and sensitivity to the differences individuals, groups, and organizations may have in their experiences and responses to the change.
- Ability to recognize differences and to identify similar patterns of responses to change among individuals, groups, and organizations.
- Avoid stereotyping by acknowledging variations among individuals, groups, and organizations.

> A transformative teacher is one who models caring to his or her students at all times in order for the students to reflect on themselves as caring people (Diekelmann, 1995).

- Awareness that communication is inextricably interwoven with culture.
- Awareness of how language (preference, level of comfort, proficiency) influences an individual's perception, ability to understand, develop meanings, and make sense out of their world.
- "Knowledge of diversity in communication patterns, styles, and protocols, and of how language and communication may influence the development of trust in relationships" (Meleis, 1999, p. 12).

## Strategies for Planned Change

Successful change involves making a compelling case for the change and then putting into place measures to manage change risk to protect the organization and its stakeholders (Kee & Newcomer, 2008).

Strategies for leading change include:

1. "Diagnosing change risk and organizational capacity
2. Strategizing and making the case for change
3. Implementing and sustaining change
4. Reinforcing change by creating a change-centric learning organization" (p. 5)

Strom (2001) identifies the top eight effective implementation strategies:

1. *Multiple interventions:* Comprehensive interventions that take into account the many characteristics of the organization as well as the external environment.
2. *Outreach visits:* Intensive support by a change agent who provides education, feedback, practical support, reminders, and praise for progress.
3. *Opinion leaders:* Recruit individuals who are recognized by peers as influential educators to promote the change.
4. *Reminders:* Prompt health care professionals to perform a patient-specific clinical action (behavioral approach), which is generally effective across a range of clinical behaviors; this is less effective if used for routine items of care or if too many prompts are presented at the same time.
5. *Feedback:* Auditing and providing feedback of summarized clinical performance.
6. *Interactive* (computer-based): Using computer information systems to support practice, such as teleconferencing, chat room techniques, and information sharing through listservs.
7. *Interactive* (educational): Customized, phased, educational interventions designed specifically to mitigate potential barriers, including user resistance and teaching new skills.
8. *Administrative intervention CQI:* Clinical effectiveness and successful change can be achieved by using a CQI or quality management approach, focusing on the core processes as the centerpiece of the initiative (Strom, 2001).

## Clinical Faculty Orientation

The current nursing shortage is compounded by the even greater nursing faculty shortage. The American Association of Colleges of Nursing (AACN) issued a statement warning that:

> faculty shortages at nursing schools across the country are limiting student capacity at a time when the need for nurses continues to grow. Budget constraints, an aging faculty, and increasing job competition from clinical sites have contributed to this emerging crisis (American Association of Colleges of Nursing [AACN], 2004, p. 1).

This realization has resulted in efforts on the part of nursing school administrators to recruit faculty from the nursing workforce particularly to fill the clinical faculty role. The National League of Nursing urges caution when recruiting new faculty.

> The academic community also should not assume that individuals learn to be teachers, advisors, curriculum developers, and educational leaders through "on-the-job training" or "trial by fire," rather than through planned, deliberate preparation for such roles and responsibilities. The concepts of *excellence as a teacher or excellence as a faculty member* must be discussed more often in the academic community, and more attention must be given to the ongoing development of faculty as educators (NLN, 2002, p. 3).

In lieu of formal education in the nurse educator role, a structured training program should be in place to help with the transition. The NLN recommends that pro-active measures by individual nurses and faculty be taken to support the development of the next generation of nursing educators. This includes recommendations that:

- "Nurses should seek out and take advantage of opportunities that prepare them for a nurse educator role
- Faculty should promote careers in nursing education through the early identification of talented neophytes and the encouragement of experienced nurses who have demonstrated nurse educator skills
- Senior faculty who, themselves, are expert educators should mentor novices and foster their professional growth in the role" (NLN, 2002, p. 4).

## Evidence-Based Education

Wardell (2007) compared the use of Chickering and Gamson's (1987) seven principles of good teaching with associate professors who taught in nursing programs ($N = 252$). The study found that experienced faculty with formal educational training scored significantly better in three of the seven principles when compared with faculty with less experience and no formal educational courses. Those three principles were student-faculty contact, active learning, and expectations of students.

The Montgomery College Nursing Program, in Maryland, identifies critical areas of performance for clinical faculty. These include:

- *Problem Solving/Critical Thinking:* Encourages critical thinking and initiative among students, provides assistance when needed.
- *Clinical Performance/Competency:* Participates in continuing education activities on a regular basis; demonstrates depth of knowledge in the clinical setting; is prepared and organized in the clinical setting.

■ *Communication:* Provides a non-threatening learning environment; communicates expectations; identifies student strengths and weaknesses; documents areas for improvement.

■ *Leadership:* Expects professional accountability; acts as a liaison between clinical facility, college, and students; models ethical nursing practice.

■ *Integrating:* Discusses clinical experience in lights of Holism and related theories; conducts pre and post conferences according to course objectives; assigns clinical activities to meet individual learning needs and course objectives.

It is essential that clinical faculty are provided training and support to achieve these performance criteria and to become familiar with the educator role. Several schools of nursing have introduced innovative approaches to address the learning needs of new clinical educators. For example, Indiana University School of Nursing has a Web-based course entitled "Clinical Faculty: A New Practice Role" that allows novice clinical faculty to "become familiar with content related to the role of a clinical educator, including scenarios, resources, and examples for the nurse who is responsible for the clinical supervision and evaluation of nursing students or staff in a health care facility" (Indiana University School of Nursing, 2009, para. 1). The course provides the learner the opportunity to "discuss role development, managing the clinical day, clinical instruction and evaluation, policies and procedures, and strategies to support and encourage student learning" (Indiana University School of Nursing, 2009, para. 1). Course objectives include:

1. "Identifying policies, procedures, and resources to fulfill the clinical teaching role
2. Recognizing the roles of clinical educator
3. Describing strategies to guide, support, facilitate, and encourage student learning
4. Identifying the multiple components necessary to organize and implement the activities related to a clinical day
5. Listing guidelines for documenting student progress on clinical evaluation tools
6. Using effective evaluation principles when giving students feedback about clinical performance
7. Describing the interplay of student, environment, teaching, and evaluation in clinical education
8. Developing an online network to share teaching and learning knowledge and experiences" (Indiana University School of Nursing, 2009, para. 1).

Approximately two to four objectives are appropriate for an hour of classroom instruction.

Another example of an innovative approach to supporting the learning needs of novice clinical faculty is offered by Drexel University's College of Nursing and Health Professions. This program offers:

- Structured face-to-face orientation
- Ongoing Web-based training and support via a course management system (Blackboard) that supports"just-in-time" tutorials, which are available 24/7.
- A course-based Clinical Communication Center that facilitates communication between course and clinical faculty helping to bridge the gap between classroom and clinical learning.
- An annual day-long faculty development workshop to build educator skills
- Dedicated clinical faculty liaisons and mentorship
- Quarterly technology workshops

## Interfacing With the Larger Academic Community and Administration

### Collaborator Role of the Nurse Educator

Collaborating with the larger academic community, administration, and the external community is an important role for the nurse educator. The ability to interact effectively with diverse entities and form collaborative partnerships is an essential in efforts to provide optimal educational opportunities for the next generation of nurses.

- In these efforts, the nurse educator needs to apply specific core "knowledge and skills associated with collaboration to enact and enhance the best practices for the teacher and scholar roles" (Southern Regional Education Board [SREB], 2002, p. 9).
- Green (2006) states that nurse educators in health care organizations often play key roles in collaborative initiatives utilizing collaboration skills to form alliances [of] nursing faculty in academia to better use resources in order to improve and expand learning outcomes.
- These collaborative teams have found innovative ways to accomplish needed research, develop curricula, and accommodate the nursing shortage to mutually benefit both service and academic institutions. (p. 282)

The Southern Regional Education Board (2002) has identified specific core knowledge and skills for collaboration and detailed collaboration competencies. Core knowledge and skills consist of:

- "Knowledge of relevant theories (group, leadership, communication, negotiation, organization, systems, change)
- Problem-solving/decision-making skills
- Knowledge of legislative and policy development processes.

Expected competencies for the collaborator role include" (SREB, 2002, p. 9):

- Consult with others within and outside of the discipline
- Establish strong links among educational institutions, clinical institutions and the community

- Use broad frameworks to build effective relationships within and among groups to enhance nursing education
- Communicate effectively with peers, students, administrators, communities and others to facilitate the enactment of best practices in nursing education
- Work with others to promote nursing and health care in political or legislative agendas
- Explain the nursing curriculum to various constituencies—peers, students, administrators, regulatory agencies and other health-related disciplines
- Demonstrate professional and educational values and legal/ethical precepts in interactions.

The Community-Campus Partnerships for Health (CCPH) is an organization that has been in existence since 1996 with the mission to "foster partnerships between communities and educational institutions that build on each other's strengths and develop their roles as change agents for improving health professions education, civic responsibility and the overall health of communities" (Community-Campus Partnerships for Health [CCPH], 2009, para. 1). This organization's *Principles of Good Community-Campus Partnerships* can provide

| Exhibit 6.1 | Principles of Good Community-Campus Partnerships |
|---|---|

- Partners have agreed upon the mission, values, goals, and measurable outcomes for the partnership.
- The relationship between partners is characterized by mutual trust, respect, genuineness, and commitment.
- The partnership builds upon identified strengths and assets, but also addresses areas that need improvement.
- The partnership balances power among partners and enables resources to be shared among partners.
- There is clear, open and accessible communication between partners who make it an ongoing priority to listen to each other's needs, develop a common language, and validate/clarify the meaning of terms.
- Roles, norms, and processes for the partnership are established with the input and agreement of all partners.
- There is feedback to, among, and from all stakeholders in the partnership, with the goal of continuously improving the partnership and its outcomes.
- Partners share the credit for the partnership's accomplishments.
- Partnerships take time to develop and evolve over time.

From 2008 Community-Campus Partnerships for Health c/o Medical College of Wisconsin, Public and Community Health, Retrieved December 14, 2008, from http://depts.washington.edu/ccph/principles.html#principles

a framework for establishing mutually beneficial collaborative partnerships (see Exhibit 6.1).

## Strategies for Improving University-Community Collaboration

Effective communication is central to any successful university-community collaboration. The primary reason that university-community partnerships fail is due to a lack of communication and a lack of an identified contact person within each partner organization (Walsh, 2006). Successful university-community collaborations require considerable time and effort from all parties. Coalition-building is a process that requires building trust, creating a shared vision, and providing a service (Erwin, Blumenthal, Chapel, & Allwood, 2004).

Essential ingredients for successful academic-community partnerships identified by Plowfield, Wheeler, and Raymond (2005) include time, tact, talent, and trust.

- *Time* must be invested by the teacher to establish the relationship with the agency or community service being utilized. Connections have to be established person to person and electronically to understand the needs of both groups and the resources available. Time is also a detriment to the process because establishing a service-learning curriculum is time-intensive for faculty, who are already overextended.
- *Tact* is necessary to ensure a trusting relationship. Communication is a key element, as is maintaining the vision of the project throughout the process of detail analysis. Tact calls for respect, which means prompt answers, attending to matters, answering questions, and anticipating problems.
- *Talent* is recognizing and celebrating different areas of expertise in situations. Plowfield, Wheeler, and Raymond (2005) state, "No one wants to invest time and resources when objectives are not clear or the path to achieving them is fraught with obstacles" (p. 219). Talent guards against this pitfall in service learning.
- *Trust-building* is an ongoing process, forged through the other three values in a service-learning project. Trust is built through open dialogue and tact while working together on mutual goals (Plowfield et al., 2005).

Erwin et al. have also identified three "lessons learned" as being potentially useful to other institutions or organizations that are attempting to develop partnerships:

1. "Work hard to establish trust and a shared sense that all the partners are committed to a common goal. These two characteristics represent the *sine qua non* without which no partnership can succeed.
2. Minimize hassles—If the "hassle factor" grows large enough, partners may decide that it would be better to go it alone.
3. Ensure that each partner receives a tangible benefit from the partnership. This could be in the form of funding, personnel, or services" (p. 601).

## Partnerships to Expand the Learning Environment

In this era of financial constraints and shrinking resources, academic organizations must seek innovative solutions to meet the education needs of their students. The AACN (2005) suggests strategies that can be utilized to expand the learning environment. These include:

1. "Increase formal partnerships between schools of nursing and clinical facilities, identifying and capitalizing on specific benefits that are attractive and useful to both partners.
2. Develop clinical faculty appointments or other forms of recognition/inducement to qualified clinical agency personnel in return for their supervising/teaching students in those agencies.
3. As needed, educate agency personnel regarding strategies for clinical teaching and evaluation.
4. Include appropriate clinical agency personnel on school of nursing committees and task forces to gain their pragmatic perspective on the education of students.
5. Import clinical education strategies from other health disciplines, both internal and external to one's own setting, that demonstrate a faculty-sparing effect.
6. Explore use of virtual reality/simulated clinical experiences in supervised learning resource centers to reduce demands on clinical faculty" (AACN, 2005, pp. 19–20). Many organizations have formed collaborative networks to share limited resources. Examples include a consortium formed by 10 long-term care providers and three universities to permit professional and paraprofessional training. Advantages included being able to repeat programs, extending subjects of in-service education, developing network of training consultants, and promoting effective communication about regulation changes (Nahemow et al., 1998).
7. Develop formal, mutually beneficial, partnerships with clinical facilities to use expert clinicians to teach students and thereby increase faculty capacity.

   ■ Non-salaried faculty appointments (with indirect rewards) are often offered to agency clinicians who serve as teachers and/or clinical preceptors for students
   ■ Agency benefits:

      ■ Faculty services such as teaching or consultation
      ■ Preferred placement of employees in the academic program
      ■ Collaboration as they seek magnet recognition and similar status from external agencies;
      ■ Priority in recruiting the school's students upon graduation

8. Simulation labs:

   ■ The benefits of simulation as an alternative means for providing essential clinical experience to students are well documented in the literature.
   ■ However, the costs associated with establishing simulation facilities, even on a limited basis, remain prohibitive for many agencies or academic institutions.
   ■ Partnerships between academic institutions and health care agencies can help manage costs through sharing of resources.

- "Partnerships between clinical settings and schools of nursing to allow sharing of laboratory resources are developing in most parts of the country, though there are still many barriers to overcome. These barriers include:

  - Lack of operations experts
  - Incorporating human simulation into individualized teaching scenarios is time intensive
  - Lack of adequate staff and faculty resources to facilitate requests for assistance in designing simulations, teaching students, and helping with scenarios and debriefings in the laboratory
  - Organizational territorialism and fear of damage to expensive resources (Gant, 2007, p. 70).

Nurse educators have a responsibility to participate in the political process to advance nursing's agenda and to advocate for nursing and nursing education (Green, 2006). Nurse educators must also integrate political processes into their practice and educational endeavors by serving as role models for the next generation of nurses. Nursing educators have both the opportunity and responsibility to advance nursing's agenda though a variety of activities (Mahoney, 2001):

- Nurturing the political involvement of student nurses and nurses who have returned to school for baccalaureate or graduate education.

  - Role modeling
  - Structured activities within the curriculum to enhance political or professional activity (including joining professional organizations, active participation on committees, and involvement in the political process)

- Development of professional nurse behaviors among students

  - Students must be empowered so that they can assume a leadership role in the setting in which they choose to practice.
  - Provide clinical experiences that develop independence and the leadership skills essential for negotiation, case management, and managed care within a complex health care environment.

- Provide opportunities for students to:

  - Become aware of the issues affecting health care
  - Develop an understanding of ethical issues in a climate of shrinking health care resources
  - Identify opportunities to influence change

In *The Essentials of Baccalaureate Education for Professional Nursing Practice*, the American Association of Colleges of Nursing (AACN, 2008) identifies core educational outcomes for undergraduate nursing education in relation to health care policy, finance, and regulatory environments. The AACN maintains that "healthcare policies, including financial and regulatory, directly and indirectly influence the nature and functioning of the healthcare system and thereby are important considerations in professional nursing practice" (2008, p. 3). See Exhibit 6.2.

| Exhibit 6.2 | Essential V: Healthcare Policy, Finance, and Regulatory Environments |
|---|---|

Rationale:

Health care policies, including financial and regulatory policies, directly and indirectly influence nursing practice and the nature and functioning of the health care system.

These policies shape responses to organizational, local, national, and global issues of equity, access, affordability, and social justice in health care. Health care policies also are central to any discussion about quality and safety in the practice environment.

The Baccalaureate-educated graduate will have a solid understanding of the broader context of health care, including how patient care services are organized and financed, and how reimbursement is structured. Regulatory agencies define boundaries of nursing practice, and graduates need to understand the scope and role of these agencies.

Baccalaureate graduates will also understand how health care issues are identified, how health care policy is both developed and changed, and how that process can be influenced through the efforts of nurses and other health care professionals, as well as lay and special advocacy groups.

Health care policy shapes the nature, quality, and safety of the practice environment and all professional nurses have the responsibility to participate in the political process and advocate for patients, families, communities, the nursing profession, and changes in the health care system, as needed. Advocacy for vulnerable populations with the goal of promoting social justice is also recognized as moral and ethical responsibilities of the nurse.

A Baccalaureate program prepares a graduate to:

1. Demonstrate basic knowledge of health care policy, finance, and regulatory environments, including local, state, national, and global health care trends.
2. Describe how health care is organized and financed, including the implications of business principles, such as patient and system cost factors.
3. Compare the benefits and limitations of the major forms of reimbursement on the delivery of health care services.
4. Examine legislative and regulatory processes relevant to the provision of health care.
5. Describe state and national statutes, rules, and regulations that authorize and define professional nursing practice.
6. Explore the impact of sociocultural, economic, legal, and political factors influencing health care delivery and practice.
7. Examine the roles and responsibilities of the regulatory agencies and their effect on patient care quality, workplace safety, and the scope of nursing and other health professionals' practice.

*(Continued)*

| Exhibit 6.2 | Essential V: Healthcare Policy, Finance, and Regulatory Environments (Continued) |
|---|---|

8. Discuss the implications of health care policy on issues of access, equity, affordability, and social justice in health care delivery.
9. Use an ethical framework to evaluate the impact of social policies on health care, especially for vulnerable populations.
10. Articulate, through a nursing perspective, issues concerning health care delivery to decision makers within health care organizations and other policy arenas. Participate as a nursing professional in political processes and grassroots legislative efforts to influence health care policy.
11. Advocate for consumers and the nursing profession.

Sample Content:

- Policy development and the legislative process
- Policy development and the regulatory process
- Licensure and regulation of nursing practice
- Social policy/public policy
- Policy analysis and evaluation
- Health care financing and reimbursement
- Economics of health care
- Consumerism and advocacy
- Political activism and professional organizations
- Disparities in the health care system
- The impact of social trends such as genetics and genomics, childhood obesity, and aging on health policy
- Role of nurse as patient advocate
- Ethical and legal issues
- Professional organizations' role in health care policy, finance and regulatory environments
- Scope of practice and policy perspectives of other health professionals
- Negligence, malpractice, and risk management
- Nurse Practice Act

From "The Essentials of Baccalaureate Education for Professional Nursing Practice," by American Association of Colleges of Nursing, 2008. Retrieved December 13, 2008, from http://www.aacn.nche.edu/Education/pdf/BaccEssentials08.pdf

## Political Action Resources

- Professional organizations (e.g., AACN, NLN, etc.)
- Political organizations (e.g., American Civil Liberties Union [ACLU])
- Federal, state, and local government agencies (e.g., Occupational Safety and Health Administration [OSHA])

- Electronic political information organizations (e.g., Electronic News Media, Political Information Search Engine [http://www.politicalinformation.com], etc.)
- Government representatives (e.g., contact federal, state, and local representatives via USA.gov Web sites such as http://www.usa.gov/Contact/Elected.shtml)

## Service Learning

Service learning gets students out into the community in the form of a partnership. The students learn from the experience as they provide a needed service to humanity. Service learning encourages interaction, caring, and dialogue; a service-learning project can be integrated into a curriculum as an assignment. Service learning supports the development of cultural awareness and sensitivity but does not count toward clinical hours. Vanderhoff (2005) defines service learning as "giving students the opportunity to provide service to others while tying in learning objectives and a class project for professional development" (p. 36).

### Characteristics of Service Learning

- Almost 30% of the 6.7 million students in public and private four-year college settings participate in a course in which service learning is integrated into the curriculum (National Service Learning Clearinghouse, 2004). In addition, about 50% of community colleges offer service learning courses throughout many disciplines (National Service Learning Clearinghouse, 2004). Service learning is more than volunteerism because students generally receive a percentage of their grade in response to the learning activity.
- Service learning may take place in local, community-based settings, or even internationally (Perry & Mander, 2005).
- Service learning entails recognizing the needs of the community or a given patient population (Vanderhoff, 2005).
- Service learning develops cultural competency among students through reflection and the discussion of real life experiences.
- Service learning develops collaboration skills among students. A cooperative purpose is always a powerful tool in education.

### Faculty and Institutional Roles in Service Learning

Faculty involvement in service learning is critical because, in its most common form, service learning is a course-driven feature of the curriculum. Therefore, it is important that faculty become involved at an advisory committee level in any service learning initiative.

The academic organization must be committed to the service learning initiative. A mechanism of support for faculty must be in place to:

- Generate interest among faculty in service learning
- Provide faculty with support to make the curricular changes necessary to add a service learning component to a course

An overview of faculty and institutional activities that support service learning are presented in Exhibit 6.3.

| Exhibit 6.3 | Examples of Institutional and Faculty Activities That Support Service Learning | |
|---|---|---|
| | Institution | Faculty |
| Planning | ■ Form a planning group of key persons<br>■ Survey institutional resources and climate<br>■ Attend Campus Compact Regional Institute<br>■ Develop a Campus Action Plan for service learning<br>■ Form an advisory committee | ■ Survey faculty interest and service learning courses currently offered<br>■ Identify faculty for a service learning planning group and advisory committee |
| Awareness | ■ Inform key administrators and faculty groups about service learning and program development<br>■ Join national organizations (e.g., Campus Compact, National Society for Experiential Education, Partnership for Service-Learning)<br>■ Attend service learning conferences | ■ Distribute information on service learning (e.g., brochures, newsletters, and articles)<br>■ Identify a faculty liaison in each academic unit |
| Prototype | ■ Identify and consult with exemplary programs in higher education | ■ Identify or develop prototype course(s) |
| Resources | ■ Obtain administrative commitments for an Office of Service Learning (e.g., budget, office space, personnel) | ■ Identify interested faculty and faculty mentors<br>■ Maintain syllabus file by discipline |

*(Continued)*

| Exhibit 6.3 | Examples of Institutional and Faculty Activities That Support Service Learning (Continued) | |

| | Institution | Faculty |
| --- | --- | --- |
| | ■ Develop a means for coordinating service learning with other programs on campus (e.g., student support services, faculty development) <br> ■ Apply for grants | ■ Compile a library collection on service learning <br> ■ Secure faculty development funds for expansion <br> ■ Identify existing resources that can support faculty development in service learning <br> ■ Establish a faculty award that recognizes service |
| Expansion | ■ Discuss service learning with a broader audience of administrators and staff (e.g., deans, counselors, student affairs) <br> ■ Support attendance at service learning conferences <br> ■ Collaborate with others in programming and grant applications <br> ■ Arrange campus speakers and forums on service learning | ■ Offer faculty development workshops <br> ■ Arrange one-on-one consultations <br> ■ Discuss service learning with departments and schools <br> ■ Provide course development stipends and grants to support service learning <br> ■ Focus efforts on underrepresented schools <br> ■ Develop faculty mentoring program <br> ■ Promote the development of general education, sequential, and interdisciplinary service learning courses |
| Recognition | ■ Publicize the university's service learning activities to other institutions <br> ■ Participate in conferences and workshops <br> ■ Publish research <br> ■ Publicize service learning activities in local media | ■ Publicize faculty accomplishments <br> ■ Include service learning activities on faculty annual report forms <br> ■ Involve faculty in professional activities (e.g., publications, workshops, conferences, forums) <br> ■ Publicize recipients of the faculty service award |

*(Continued)*

| Exhibit 6.3 | Examples of Institutional and Faculty Activities That Support Service Learning (Continued) |
|---|---|

**Monitoring**
- Collect data within the institution (e.g., number of courses, number of faculty teaching service learning courses, number of students enrolled, number of agency partnerships)
- Collect data on faculty involvement (e.g., number of faculty involved in faculty development activities, number of faculty offering service learning courses)

**Evaluation**
- Compile annual report for the Office of Service Learning
- Include service learning in institutional assessments
- Provide assessment methods and designs to faculty (e.g., peer review, portfolios)
- Evaluate course outcomes (e.g., student satisfaction, student learning)

**Research**
- Conduct research on service learning within the institution and across institutions
- Facilitate faculty research on service learning
- Conduct research on faculty involvement in service learning

**Institutionalization**
- Service is part of the university mission statement and service learning is recognized in university publications
- Service learning is an identifiable feature of general education
- Service learning courses are listed in bulletins, schedules of classes, and course descriptions
- University sponsors regional or national conferences on service learning
- Hard-line budget commitments to sustain service learning programs
- Service learning is part of personnel decisions (e.g., hiring, annual reviews, promotion, and tenure)
- Service learning is a permanent feature of course descriptions and the curriculum
- Service learning is an integral part of the faculty's professional development program

Adapted from "Implementing Service Learning in Higher Education," by R. G. Bringle and J. A. Hatcher, 1996. *Journal of Higher Education, 67*(2).

# CASE STUDIES

## Case Study 6.1

St. Mary's Hospital, a mid-sized community hospital, initiated a hospital-wide clinical improvement project. An interdisciplinary team of health care professionals was recruited to serve on the clinical improvement project panel. One area identified for improvement was to reduce the number of patient falls. A comprehensive, 40-page clinical guideline published by the U.S. Agency for Health Care Research and Quality (AHRQ) was selected for implementation, however the project team determined that full implementation of these guidelines was too complex and time consuming for the staff, and therefore would not likely be successful. The panel identified two changes that could be easily implemented and would likely have a significant impact on fall incident rates. A nurse representative from each in-patient unit was recruited to serve as unit leader for the implementation of these changes. A targeted information campaign was designed, and staff in-services were conducted on all units for all shifts. Those two simple innovations, not the larger, more detailed and complex guideline, reduced the rate of falls in vulnerable patients by 75%.

What strategies for change were utilized by the panel to implement this clinical improvement project? How was Rogers's Theory of Diffusion applied? How would the principles of leadership support the process? How can Scott's evaluation criteria for organizational effectiveness be applied in this scenario? Which criteria would be relevant?

## Case Study 6.2

The Nursing Programs of Drexel University, the Community College of Philadelphia, Bloomsburg University of Pennsylvania, and Howard University entered into a collaborative agreement to incorporate the use of technology in their respective undergraduate and graduate nursing programs. Drexel University, College of Nursing and Health Professions (DUCNHP), with Dr. Linda Wilson as the project director, will be the lead school and will share its technology expertise and resources by working jointly with the faculty of the collaborating schools to ensure faculty competence in selected technologies used by DUCNHP to enhance nursing education curricula and teaching processes. Topics that fall under this initiative include the following: "incorporation of the Personal Digital Assistant in didactic courses and in clinical, development, and implementation of cases and evaluation methods for Human Simulation including the use of standardized patients and patient simulators, use of Web-based courseware, and development of a server repository/portal for various interactive learning modules for use by the collaborating nursing programs" (Wilson, 2007, p. 1).

How can the principles of good community-campus partnerships be applied to this initiative to increase the likelihood of success? What strategies for change must be considered? Discuss this initiative from the perspective of organizational culture. What factors must be considered?

## Practice Questions

1. Scott (1996) states that the first step in evaluating effectiveness of an organization is:
   A. Focus on materials that the organization has developed
   B. Assess efforts made by the organization
   C. Establish standards to use for comparison
   D. Identify organizational features or characteristics

2. An indicator for evaluating the organizational effectiveness of a school of nursing from a structural perspective includes:
   A. Number of students graduated
   B. Number of students passing the NCLEX-RN
   C. Employee satisfaction
   D. Faculty characteristics and qualifications

3. An indicator for evaluating the organizational effectiveness of a school of nursing from an outcome perspective includes:
   A. Clinical lab facilities
   B. Number of students passing the NCLEX-RN
   C. Faculty characteristics and qualifications
   D. Number of research awards granted

4. An individual's perception of an organization's openness to creativity is influenced by the presence of interactional factors such as:
   A. Intellectual orientation
   B. Work load
   C. Organizational infrastructure
   D. Financial resources

5. An individual's willingness to initiate creative efforts is influenced by:
   A. Organizational stability
   B. Organizational openness
   C. Organizational structure
   D. Organizational capacity

6. Lewin's change theory is characterized by the presence of:
   A. The motivation and capacity for change
   B. Driving and restraining forces
   C. Self-efficacy
   D. Perceived control over opportunities

7. The Theory of Reasoned Action is characterized by the presence of:
   A. The motivation and capacity for change
   B. Self-efficacy
   C. Intention to perform an action
   D. Perceived control over opportunities

8. Lippitt's Phases of Change theory is characterized by the presence of:
   A. The motivation and capacity for change
   B. Self-efficacy
   C. Intention to perform an action
   D. Perceived control over opportunities

9. An example of a faculty activity that supports recognition for service learning activities is:
   A. Offering faculty development workshops
   B. Identifying a faculty liaison in each academic unit
   C. Involving faculty in opportunities for publication
   D. Collecting data on faculty involvement in service learning

10. An example of an institutional activity that supports planning for service learning activities is:
    A. Publicize service learning activities
    B. Form an advisory committee
    C. Join national service learning organizations
    D. Arrange for campus forum on service learning

## References

American Association of Colleges of Nursing (AACN). (2004). Nursing faculty shortage fact sheet. Retrieved December 13, 2008, from http://www.aacn.nche.edu/Media/Background ers/facultyshortage.htm

American Association of Colleges of Nursing (AACN). (2005). Faculty shortages in baccalaureate and graduate nursing programs: Scope of the problem and strategies for expanding the supply. Retrieved December 13, 2008, from http://www.aacn.nche.edu/Media/Back grounders/facultyshortage.htm

American Association of Colleges of Nursing (AACN). (2008). The essentials of baccalaureate education for professional nursing practice. Retrieved December 13, 2008, from http://www.aacn.nche.edu/Education/pdf/BaccEssentials08.pdf

Bass, B. (1990). From transactional to transformational leadership: learning to share the vision. *Organizational Dynamics, 18*(3), 19–31.

Bentley, R., & Ellison, K. (2005). Impact of a service-learning project on nursing students. *Nursing Education Perspectives, 26*(5), 287–290.

Berwick, D. M. (2003). Disseminating innovations in health care. *Journal of the American Medical Association, 289*(15), 1969–1975.

Bringle, R. G., & Hatcher, J. A. (1996). Implementing service learning in higher education. *Journal of Higher Education, 67*(2), 67–73.

Carroll, T. L. (2005). Leadership skills and attributes of women and nurse executives. *Nurse Administrator, 29*(2), 146–153.

Cheng, Y. C., (1996). *School effectiveness and school-based management: A mechanism for development.* London: Routledge.

Chickering, A.W., & Gamson, Z.F. (March 1987). Seven principles for good practice in undergraduate education. *American Association for Higher Education Bulletin,* 3–7.

Clark, D. R. (2008). Concepts of Leadership. Retrieved December 10, 2008, from http://www.nwlink.com/~donclark/leader/leadcon.html

Community-Campus Partnerships for Health (CCPH). (2009). Retrieved April 2, 2009, from http://www.ccph.info/

Dickenson-Hazard, N. (2004). Notes from the chief executive officer. "I have experienced this before." *Reflections on Nursing Leadership, 30*(2), 4, 38.

Diekelmann, N. L. (1995). Reawakening thinking: Is traditional pedagogy nearing completion? *Journal of Nursing Education, 34*(5), 195–196.

Ekvall, G., & Ryhammer, L. (1999). The creative climate: Its determinants and effects at a Swedish university. *Creative Research Journal, 12,* 303–310.

Erwin, K., Blumenthal, D. S., Chapel, T., & Allwood, L. V. (2004). Building an academic-community partnership for increasing the representation of minorities in the health professions. *Journal of Health Care for the Poor and Underserved, 15*(4), 589–602. Retrieved December 9, 2008, from Research Library Core database (Document ID: 736165141).

Gant, L. T. (2007). Human Simulation in Emergency Nursing Education: Current Status. *Journal of Emergency Nursing, 33*(1), 69–71.

Glasgow, M. E. S., & Cornelius F. H. (2005). Benefits and costs of integration of technology into an undergraduate nursing program. *Nursing Leadership Forum, 9*(4),175.

Green, D. A. (2006). A synergy model of nursing education. *Journal for Nurses in Staff Development, 22*(6), 277–283.

Grenny, J., Maxfield, D., & Shimberg, A, (2008). How to have influence. *MIT Sloan Management Review, 50*(1), 47–52. Retrieved December 9, 2008, from Business Module database (Document ID: 1570723531).

Grizzell, J. (2007). Behavior change theories and models. Retrieved December 14, 2007, from http://www.csupomona.edu/%7Ejvgrizzell/best_practices/bctheory.html#Reasoned%20 Action

Indiana University School of Nursing. (2009). *Clinical faculty a new practice role.* Retrieved April 3, 2009, from http://nursing.iupui.edu/continuing/courses/clinicalfaculty.shtml

Kee, J. E., & Newcomer, K. E. (2008). Why do change efforts fail? *Public Manager, 37*(3), 5–12. Retrieved December 9, 2008, from *Social Science Module Database* (Document ID: 1592581511).

Kritsonis, A. (2004–2005). Comparison of change theories. *International Journal of Scholarly Academic Intellectual Diversity, 8*(1). Retrieved December 14, 2008, from http://www.national forum.com/Electronic%20Journal%20Volumes/Kritsonis,%20Alicia%20Comparison%20 of%20Change%20Theories.pdf

Longest, B. B. (1998). Managerial competence at senior levels of integrated delivery systems. *Journal of Healthcare Management, 43*(2). 115.

Mahoney, J. (2001). Leadership skills for the 21st century. *Nursing Management, 9*(5), 269–271.

Martin, J., & Meyerson, D. (1988). Organizational culture and the denial: channeling and acknowledgement of ambiguity. In L. Pondy, R. Boland, & H. Thomas (Eds.), *Managing ambiguity and change* (pp. 93–125). New York: Wiley.

Meleis, A. I. (1999). Culturally competent care. *Journal of Transcultural Nursing, 10*(1), 12.

Mumford, M. D., Connelly, S., & Gaddis, B. (2003). How creative leaders think: Experimental findings and cases. *The Leadership Quarterly, 14,* 411–432.

Mumford, M. D., Scott, G. M., Gaddis, B., & Strange, J. M. (2002). Leading creative people: Orchestrating expertise and relationships. *The Leadership Quarterly, 13,* 705–750.

Nahemow, L., Casey, J., Gauthier, B. B., Lusky, R., & Wolf, M. A. (1988). Sharing educational resources among long-term care providers. *Educational Gerontology, 14*(3), 229–235.

National League for Nursing (NLN). (2005). Core competencies of nurse educators with task statements. *National League for Nursing.* Retrieved December 24, 2008, from http://www. nln.org/facultydevelopment/pdf/corecompetencies.pdf

National League of Nursing (NLN) Board of Governors. (2002). *Position statement: The preparation of nurse educators.* Retrieved December 20, 2008, from http://www.nln.org/aboutnln/ PositionStatements/preparation051802.pdf

National Service Learning Clearinghouse. (2004). Retrieved November 28, 2005, from http:// www.servicelearning.org/index.php

Nauheimer, H. (2005). *Taking stock: A survey on the practice and future of change management.* Johannesburg, South Africa: ChangeSource.

Nelson, D., Godfrey, L., & Purdy, J. (2004). Using a Mentorship Program to Recruit and Retain Student Nurses. *Journal of Nursing Administration, 34*(12), 551–553.

Ogbonna, E., & Harris, L.C. (2000). Leadership style, organizational culture and performance: empirical evidence from UK companies. *International Journal of Human Resource Management, 11*(4), 766–788.

Perry, S., & Mander, R. (2005). A global frame of reference: learning from everyone, everywhere. *Nursing Education Perspectives, 26*(3), 148–151.

Plowfield, L., Wheeler, E., & Raymond, J. (2005). Time, tact, talent and trust: Essential ingredients of effective academic-community partnership. *Nursing Educational Perspectives, 26*(4), 217–220.

Rogers, E. M. (2003). *Diffusion of innovations* (5th ed.). New York: Free Press.

Sarros, J. C., Cooper, B. K., & Santora, J. C. (2008). Building a climate for innovation through transformational leadership and organizational culture. *Journal of Leadership & Organizational Studies, 15*(2), 145. Retrieved December 9, 2008, from Education Module database (Document ID: 1575665161).

Southern Regional Education Board (SREB). (2002). *Nurse educator competencies.* Retrieved December 10, 2008, from http.//www.sreb.org

Strom, K. (2001). Quality improvement interventions: What works? *Journal for Healthcare Quality, 23*(5), 4–14.

Thibodeaux, M. S., & Favilla, E. (1996). Organizational effectiveness and commitment through strategic management. *Industrial Management & Data Systems, 96*(5), 21–25.

Vanderhoff, M. (2005). Service learning: The world as the classroom. *PT Magazine, 13*(5), 34–41.

Walsh, D. (2006). Best practices in university-community partnerships: Lessons learned from a physical-activity-based program. *Journal of Physical Education, Recreation & Dance, 77*(4), 45–49, 56. Retrieved December 9, 2008, from Research Library Core database (Document ID: 1023544281).

Wardell, N. (2007). *The use of principles of good practice in undergraduate registered nursing programs in seven mid-western states.* Unpublished manuscript, University of Nebraska–Lincoln.

Weston, M. J., Falter, B., Lamb, G. S., Mahon, G., Malloch, K., Provan, K. G., et al. (2008). Health care leadership academy: A statewide collaboration to enhance nursing leadership competencies. *Journal of Continuing Education in Nursing, 39*(10), 468–472.

White, A. (2004). Change strategies make for smooth transitions. *Nursing Management, 35*(2), 49–52. Retrieved December 4, 2008, from ABI/INFORM Global database. (Document ID: 546126451).

Wilson, L. (2007). *Faculty development: Integrated technology into nursing education & practice.* Unpublished grant proposal, Drexel University, Philadelphia.

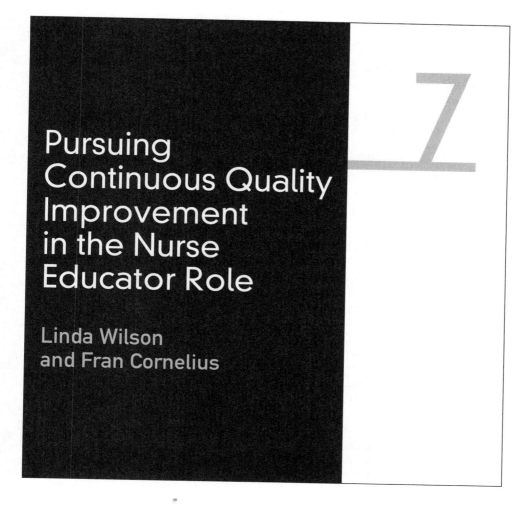

# Pursuing Continuous Quality Improvement in the Nurse Educator Role

**7**

Linda Wilson
and Fran Cornelius

*If you don't know where you are going, any road will take you there.*

—spoken by Alice, in Lewis Carroll's *Alice in Wonderland*

**NLN Core Competency VI: Pursue Continuous Quality Improvement in Nurse Educator Role**

Nurse educators recognize that their role is multidimensional and that an ongoing commitment to develop and maintain competence in the role is essential (National League for Nursing [NLN], 2005, p. 21).

**Learning Outcomes**

- Identifies activities that promote one's socialization to the nursing role
- Discuss the importance of a mentor across the career trajectory
- Discuss the importance of a commitment to lifelong learning
- Discuss the importance of membership and active participation in professional organizations

- Identifies professional development opportunities that increase one's effectiveness in the nursing role
- Discuss the importance of balancing teaching, scholarship, service and institutional demands
- Identify sources of feedback to improve role effectiveness
- Discuss the opportunities available for including technology in the learning environment
- Discuss the essential informatics competencies and strategies to incorporate into the curriculum

## Introduction

The National League of Nursing holds that nurse educators "recognize that their role is multidimensional and that an ongoing commitment to develop and maintain competence in the role is essential. To pursue continuous quality improvement in the nurse educator role, the individual:

- Demonstrates a commitment to lifelong learning
- Recognizes that career enhancement needs and activities change as experience is gained in the role
- Participates in professional development opportunities that increase one's effectiveness in the role
- Balances the teaching, scholarship, and service demands inherent in the role of educator and member of an academic institution
- Uses feedback gained from self, peer, student, and administrative evaluation to improve role effectiveness
- Engages in activities that promote one's socialization to the role
- Uses knowledge of legal and ethical issues relevant to higher education and nursing education as a basis for influencing, designing, and implementing policies and procedures related to students, faculty, and the educational environment
- Mentors and supports faculty colleagues" (NLN, 2005, p. 6).

This chapter will focus on the essential elements in the pursuit of continuous quality improvement. These include:

1. Socialization to the faculty role
2. Role of mentorship across the career continuum
3. Active membership in professional organizations
4. Commitment to lifelong learning
5. Technology and informatics in the learning environment
6. Balancing teaching, scholarship, and service
7. Self-reflection to promote professional development

## Socialization to the Educator Role

The role of a new academic nurse educator can be both exciting and challenging. One of the most important support systems for a new educator is appropriate mentoring (NLN, 2006). An orientation program should include the following:

1. Introduction to key personnel
2. Introduction to other faculty members
3. A review of available resources
4. A review of the courses and their related content
5. A review of job benefits
6. A review of administrative and governance structures
7. An introduction to the culture and political environment
8. Presentations on key aspects of the curriculum
9. A review of expectations for teaching, research, and service
10. Assignment of a faculty mentor

## Mentor and Support Faculty Colleagues

Academic nurse educators have many roles and responsibilities, including the responsibility of mentoring. Nursing faculty have a responsibility to mentor colleagues, assisting them in their development as both educators and scholars (Billings & Halstead, 2005). Faculty mentorship includes guiding, coaching, and supporting faculty as they advance in their careers. Mentoring is extremely important, particularly for novices, because graduate school often provides little preparation for the academic nurse educator role. Mentoring is also important throughout all career stages.

### Mentoring Throughout the Career Continuum

The NLN's (2006) position statement regarding *Mentoring of Nurse Faculty* highlights key mentoring activities beneficial at various stages of a nurse educator's career. These include:

- Early Career Faculty Members
  Mentorship targets the faculty member who is new to both the educator role and the institution. Mentoring

  - Helps the uninitiated learn the complexities of the faculty role.
  - Provides information about the knowledge, skills, behaviors, and values that comprise the faculty role.
  - Formal orientation programs, which often include:

    - An introduction to key personnel and resources
    - A review of the courses and curricula being taught
    - An overview of job benefits and administrative and governance structures
    - An introduction to the culture and political environment of the institution

  - An assigned mentor throughout the entire first year should:

    - Answer questions
    - Interpret situations

- Provide direct help
- Share a similar schedule to ensure optimum availability
- Be friendly and caring

- Mid-Career Faculty Members
  Mentorship supports faculty as they identify and test innovative pedagogies, propose new solutions to problems, and evolve as educator/ scholars in local, regional, and national arenas.

  - Mentoring is:

    - Eclectic, varied in its content and process
    - Directed more by the mentee than by the mentor
    - Involves reciprocal sharing, learning, and growth
    - Individually focused and takes time to evolve

  - Faculty may select a mentor for:

    - Formal and informal mentoring relationships
    - Shared interests inside and outside their academic communities
    - Development of specific aspects of teaching, evaluation of learning, curriculum design, scholarship, service, and leadership
    - Guidance in transitioning into academic leadership positions

  - Faculty may develop "multiple mentoring partnerships, where each mentor assists them to grow in a particular area, such as grantwriting or conducting research on a particular topic" or one who can "provide guidance in selecting and transitioning into academic leadership positions" (NLN, 2006, p. 4).

- Late Career Faculty Members
  At the foundation of mentorship at this level, the responsibility is to "identify new faculty members who show potential as leaders in nursing and nursing education and enter into mentor-protégé relationships with them, relationships that extend over long periods of time" (NLN, 2006, p. 4). The mentoring relationship at this level:

  - Is a source of satisfaction derived from guiding another in the attaining of self-clarity, personal growth, and as the educator continues to develop his or her skills
  - Cultivates a relationship that is situated in common interests and is built upon mutual respect for one another's knowledge and talents
  - Characterized by the investment of time, effort, and caring; the identification of mutual goals; and regular, ongoing dialogue designed to ensure the accomplishment of those goals (p. 4)

In the mentor-protégé relationship, the mentor shares her/his wisdom, knowledge, and expertise; builds connections in multiple communities by introducing personal networks; and keeps open a future of possibilities for someone who is expected to make significant contributions to the profession. Through an extended relationship, the mentor nurtures leadership in the protégé. (p. 4)

- The "key variable in the success or failure of the mentoring relationship was the mentor's accessibility, both physical and emotional" (Wasburn, 2007, p. 61).
- It is important to note that mentorship is not limited to a relationship between two faculty members.
- Mentoring, in an ideal sense, involves the entire academic community. Everyone within the organization bears a responsibility to provide a supportive and welcoming environment and to foster a sense of belonging.
- An ongoing commitment to the practice of mentoring requires support from administrators and the entire nursing faculty. "Establishing a healthful work environment where collaborative peer and co-mentoring are an expectation, rather than a possibility, is the responsibility of all involved in nursing education" (Wasburn, 2007, p. 4).

The NLN recommendations for mentoring at all levels are outlined in Exhibit 7.1.

## Membership in Professional Organizations

It is important for the academic nurse educator to have membership in professional organizations. These organizations include, but are not limited to, the following:

- American Nurses Association
- State nursing organizations
- National League for Nursing
- Sigma Theta Tau International Honor Society for Nursing
- Specialty nursing organizations (American Society of Perianesthesia Nurses, Association of periOperative Registered Nurses, National Association of Orthopaedic Nurses, Oncology Nursing Society; American Association of Critical Care Nurses, etc.)
- Other related professional organizations (American Pain Society, Society for Critical Care Medicine, American Medical Informatics Association, etc.)

Membership in professional organizations provides the opportunity for knowledge enhancement, networking, and professional activities.

## Active Participation in Professional Organizations

Professional organizational membership and leadership activities are an excellent mechanism for taking an active role in determining the future of nursing. These activities are also important in satisfying the service requirements for nurse educators.

- Participate on a committee
- Participate in a special interest group

## Exhibit 7.1          NLN Recommendations for Mentoring

*For Nursing Faculty*

- Contribute to the development of a mentoring program at your institution by identifying the needs of new faculty members and the resources required to meet those needs.
- Actively participate in mentoring relationships.
- Make the teaching done by experienced faculty members more visible to new faculty.
- Be open and friendly to new faculty and identify opportunities to be a "One Minute Mentor" through brief, supportive interactions (Oermann, 2001).
- Become sensitive to existing and potential academic community practices that exclude new faculty members.
- Spend time together as a nurse faculty community, talking and listening to one another and including the new faculty members.
- Attend professional development workshops and seminars on mentoring.
- Collaborate with the dean/director/chairperson to establish a mentoring program.
- Include content on mentoring in undergraduate and graduate curricula, including how to identify and select caring colleagues with whom to work closely and how to collaborate with colleagues.

*For Deans/Directors/Chairpersons*

- Initiate and provide support for mentoring initiatives at your institution.
- Engage new, mid-career, and seasoned faculty in developing mentoring initiatives at your institution.
- Incorporate innovative strategies for mentoring new faculty members, such as the use of retired nurse educators (Bellack, 2004).
- Value the mentor role and reward faculty who actively serve in mentoring roles.
- Support the development of faculty mentors.
- Model mentoring.

*For the National League for Nursing*

- Support research on mentoring in the academic environment.
- Offer workshops and seminars on mentoring.
- Develop a mentoring toolkit.

From "Position Statement: Mentoring of Nurse Faculty," by the National League for Nursing, 2006. *Nursing Education Perspectives, 27*(2), 110–113.

■ Serve as Chair of a committee
■ Serve as Chair of a special interest group
■ Run for an office or role on the board of directors at the local, state, or national level
■ Participate on a task force
■ Volunteer to work on specific initiatives for the organization

## Commitment to Lifelong Learning/Faculty Development

According to the *ANA Scope and Standards for Nursing Professional Development* (ANA, 2000), the following are some of the beliefs that guided the development of the standards:

■ "Lifelong learning is the responsibility of the nurse and is essential to maintain and increase competence in nursing practice" (p. 1).
■ "Continuing professional nursing competence is essential to the provision of safe, quality health care to all members of society" (p. 1).
■ "The public has a right to expect continuing professional nursing competence throughout the career of the nurse" (p. 1).
■ "Self directed learning is an integral part of continuing education, staff development and academic education" (p. 2).

The *Scope and Standards* also states that the lifelong professional development of a nurse requires participation in learning activities in order to assist in the development and maintenance of competence, enhancement of practice, and support for the attainment of career goals. The academic nurse educator has a personal and professional responsibility to:

■ Seek continuing education activities to maintain competency
■ Expand knowledge and expertise in a nursing specialty.

The NLN's (2001) position statement regarding lifelong learning acknowledges that the "concept of lifelong learning for nursing faculty is complex and multi-faceted," and that learning starts in a Master's and/or Doctoral study program, but continues beyond formal education as a lifelong pursuit. Lifelong learning continues "thorough self-study and a constant inquisitiveness about the role and all its dimensions" (p. 1).

## Participation in Professional Development Opportunities to Enhance Ongoing Development

In order to maintain high quality nursing education programs, it is imperative that all faculty remain not only proficient with basic principles but also current with emerging technology and pedagogical trends. There are many different types of professional development opportunities in which the academic nurse educator can participate.

- Provider-directed, provider-paced
- The provider-directed, provider-paced educational opportunity is an activity occurring at a date and time set by the educational provider.
- Examples of provider-directed, provider-paced educational opportunities include seminars, national conferences, and Webinars.
- Provider-directed, learner-paced
- A provider-directed, learner-paced educational activity is developed by the educational provider; the activity is completed at a time convenient for or selected by the learner.
- Examples of provider-directed, learner-paced educational activities include continuing education journal articles, online continuing education modules, and continuing education programs delivered on CDs or DVDs.

  - Learner-directed activities
  - A learner directed activity is "a learning activity where the learner takes the initiative with or without the help of others, in the following activities:
    1. Diagnosing their learning needs,
    2. Formulating learning goals,
    3. Identifying human and material resources for learning,
    4. Choosing and implementing appropriate learning strategies,
    5. Evaluating learning outcomes" (ANCC, 2006, p. 74).

While similarities in learning needs exist, the elements of lifelong learning for the nurse educator vary according to:

- Type of faculty appointment:

  - Full-time, part-time, or adjunct
  - Tenure track or non–tenure track
  - Academic or service setting

- Career stages

  - The novice
  - Mid-stage
  - Senior faculty

- "The mission of a university affects the nature of expectations for the:

  - Scope of the role of faculty
  - The educator role" (NLN, 2001, p. 1)

The NLN (2001) maintains that faculty development programs should be individualized and adaptable, and should offer a wide range of topics in multiple modalities. Topics relevant to nurse educators include, but are not limited to:

- Classroom management
- Student advisement

- Student incivility
- Cultural competency
- Informatics competency
- Clinical teaching
- Clinical evaluation
- Test construction
- Developing goal statements and learning objectives
- Outcomes assessment
- Teaching/learning technologies
- Curriculum development and modification
- The accreditation process
- The faculty role as leaders in the university community
- Creative teaching strategies
- Strategies to promote critical thinking
- Strategies to integrate informatics within the curriculum

It is important to note that "no single program or approach will meet the needs of everyone, and even the most senior tenured Full Professor must never think that she/he has nothing new to learn" (NLN, 2001, p. 2).

## Keeping Up With Information and Advances in Technology

As technology progresses, academic nurse educators must keep up with its advancement. Although it may be challenging at times, as an academic nurse educator it is important to be open-minded, eager to learn, and willing to look outside of nursing for innovative ideas that will enhance the quality of nursing education. Professional and special-interest organizations offer opportunities to stay current and network. Some organizations include:

- *Educause* (http://www.educause.edu): This nonprofit association's mission is to advance higher education by promoting the intelligent use of information technology.
- *National Education Association (NEA)* (http://www2.nea.org/he/techno.html): This organization was founded in 1857 with the goal to "both elevate the character and advance the interests of teaching, promoting the cause of education in the United States" (NEA, 2007, p. 1). The NEA higher education Web site offers a forum to discuss the role of technology in education as well as an opportunity to learn about new trends.
- *Society for Applied Learning Technologies* (SALT) (http://www.salt.org): SALT is a professional society oriented toward professionals whose work requires knowledge and communication in the field of instructional technology.

In addition, there are other resources, such as Innovate (http://www.innovateonline.info), that provide faculty the opportunity to stay current with new technologies and innovations.

## Technology in the Learning Environment

The learning environment has morphed into an arena where learners are no longer passive recipients of information. Learning has become an interactive and social experience resulting in richer, more meaningful experiences for students and faculty alike. Whether in the traditional face-to-face classroom, the clinical setting, or a virtual environment, new technologies and Web 2.0 tools provide many opportunities to enhance learning far beyond the traditional "ivory towers." Brown (2006) states:

> One would also expect a form of spiral learning to evolve, initially rooted in one community but then branching out to encompass expanding interests and skills. The spiral would weave a tapestry between activities in the niche communities of interest and the core curriculum, with both serving to ground and complement the other. This new learningscape would be supported by an understanding of the interplay between the social and cognitive basis of learning, and enabled by the networked age of the 21st century. Such an educational experience would undoubtedly build a strong foundation for life-long learning in a world of accelerating change. (p. 29)

There are many opportunities to incorporate new technologies into learning. Some examples include:

- *Web-enhanced courses:* Courses can be Web-enhanced to support any curriculum. The Internet, video streaming, podcasting, and Web 2.0 tools can help to enhance any classroom activity. Some popular Web 2.0 tools include:
    - *Wikis:* a collection of Web pages that may be edited by anyone
    - *Blogs:* journal entries that are presented in reverse chronological order
    - *Social networking:* Web sites that build relationships and connections/networks, strengthening learning communities
    - *Twitter.com:* a "micro-blog" that allows users to send short text messages not exceeding 140 characters in length to their personalized homepage
    - *Podcasting or video podcasting:* A method of distributing multimedia content (lectures, discussions, etc.) via the Internet for playback on mobile devices and personal computers
- *Mobile devices* (PDAs or smartphones):
    - Classroom: The electronic resources on these devices can be used in a variety of classroom activities such as:
        - Gaming activities like Jeopardy to review class content and stimulate learners in the classroom
        - Modeling strategies to bring new evidence into practice
    - Lab/Clinical: The electronic resources on these devices may be used to:
        - Reference step-by-step instructions for a nursing procedure, such as nasogastric tube insertion or tracheostomy care

- Model point-of-care/point-of-need information access such as drug compatibility/interactions
- *Clicker technology:* also referred to as an "audience-response system," it can be used to engage the learner in the classroom and in online environments.
  - One method for incorporating this technology is to create some pre-class questions that the students can respond to using the clicker technology, and then, following the lecture, present the same questions as post-class questions to see if there is an increase in correct responses, thereby demonstrating student comprehension of the content presented.
  - Another method is to pose questions to which there may be differing opinions. Students can respond anonymously and "the stage is set to support and deepen engagement and articulation as students try to mount arguments for their position" (Brown, 2006, p. 29).
- *Simulation:* There are multiple types of simulation available for use in the lab environment. These include:
  - Computer-based simulations
  - Human patient simulator, such as SIMMAN®.
  - Human simulation using standardized patients or patient actors.
  - Key points:
    - The choice of what type of simulation to use is based on the specific content or skills being tested and the available resources. Specific cases and evaluation criteria can be developed with either type of simulation.
    - Components for designing a simulation experience are in Exhibit 7.2.

## Evidence-Based Practice

Brannan, White, and Bezanson (2008) reported that, out of 107 nursing students, the use of a human patient simulator made a positive difference in the student's ability to answer questions on a test of cognitive skills. It did not find that confidence levels were increased significantly.

To support academic nurse educators with the use of technology, a university can:

- Provide access to new learning technologies
- Offer faculty training to support the integration of new technologies into teaching

| Exhibit 7.2 | Components to Consider When Designing a Simulation Experience |
| --- | --- |

| Component To Consider | Outcome Desired |
| --- | --- |
| Identify the focus of the experience | Communicate the learning outcomes |
| Specific diagnosis for the experience | Medical diagnosis<br>Psychosocial factors |
| Specific requirements for the experience | History taking<br>Physical exam<br>Patient teaching<br>Teamwork<br>Delegation<br>Conflict resolution<br>Comprehensive experience |
| Length of time for the experience | Adequate time to complete tasks |
| Evaluation criteria for the experience | Pass/Fail<br>Specific score/grade required |
| Debriefing method to be used | Timing of the debriefing |
| Decide if there will there be student self-evaluation | Student review of video<br>Student self-evaluation paper |

■ Establish Web-based resource centers, such as Drexel University's Virtual Nursing Faculty Resource Center (Hasson, Cornelius, & Suplee, 2008).

1. The purpose of this type of resource center is to provide Web-based support.
2. "This resource center can serve as a 'one-stop shopping' area for all faculty to access not only resources but also tutorials to support 'just-in-time' training needs" (Hasson et al., 2008, p. 23).

## Informatics in the Learning Environment

The NLN (2008) "advocates for support of faculty development initiatives and innovative educational programs that address informatics preparation. This call for reform is relevant to all prelicensure and graduate nursing education programs as the informatics revolution will impact all of nursing practice" (p. 1). See Exhibit 7.3.

Key driving forces in this process include:

■ Reports and recommendations from the Institute of Medicine
■ Creation of the Office of the National Coordinator of Health Information Technology and its federal mandates

| Exhibit 7.3 | Informatics Competencies Categories |
|---|---|
| Technical Competencies | Technical competencies are related to the actual psychomotor use of computers and other technological equipment. Specific nursing informatics competencies include the ability to use selected applications in a comfortable and knowledgeable way. It is important for nurses to feel confident in their use of computers and software in the practice setting, and especially at the bedside, in order to be able to attend to the client while using these devices. |
| Utility Competencies | Utility competencies are related to the process of using computers and other technological equipment within nursing practice, education, research, and administration. Specific nursing informatics competencies include the process of applying evidenced-based practice, critical thinking, and accountability to the use of selected applications in a comfortable and knowledgeable way. |
| Leadership Competencies | Leadership competencies are related to the ethical and management issues related to using computers and other technological equipment within nursing practice, education, research, and administration. Specific nursing informatics competencies include the process of applying accountability, client privacy and confidentiality, and quality assurance in documentation to the use of selected applications in a comfortable and knowledgeable way. |

- The Technology Informatics Guiding Educational Reform (TIGER) Initiative
- The Robert Wood Johnson Foundation-funded Quality and Safety Education for Nurses (QSEN) Initiative (NLN, 2008).

## The Technology Informatics Guiding Education Reform (TIGER) Initiative

The Technology Informatics Guiding Education Reform (TIGER) Initiative is a consortium of more than 40 nursing professional organizations that "aims to enable practicing nurses and nursing students to fully engage in the unfolding digital era of health care" (TIGER Initiative, 2007, p. 3). TIGER recommendations for schools of nursing include:

- Adopt informatics competencies for all levels of nursing education (undergraduate/graduate) and practice (generalist/specialist)
- Encourage faculty to participate in development programs in informatics
- Develop a task force or committee at each school to examine the integration of informatics throughout the curriculum
- Encourage the Health Services Resources Administration's (HRSA) Division of Nursing to continue and expand its support for informatics specialty programs and faculty development
- Measure changes from baseline in informatics knowledge among nursing educators and students and among the full range of clinicians seeking continuing education
- Collaborate with industry and service partners to support faculty creativity in the design, acceptance, and adoption of informatics technology
- Develop strategies to recruit, retain, and educate current and future nurses in the areas of informatics education, practice, and research (NLN, 2008, p. 4)

## Informatics Competencies

Specific informatics competencies include, but are not limited to, computer literacy or computer skills, information literacy or the ability to retrieve information, and general informatics skills. These skills include the ability to use informatics strategies and system applications to manage data and information and the ability to process the data retrieved (Saba & McCormick, 2006). Informatics competencies for nurses are typically organized according to three proficiency levels:

1. Beginner, entry or user level,
2. Intermediate or modifier level
3. Advanced or innovator level of competency (Saba & McCormick, 2006)

## Evidence-Based Education

Staib (2003) examined teaching methods that enhance students' critical thinking activity and found that the common threads among successful approaches included:

- Creativity
- Contextual perspective of the content
- Reflection
- Open-mindedness

Some of the techniques assessed were:

- Simulation vignettes using "real life" scenarios
- Concept mapping
- Computer-assisted instruction
- Case studies

Informatics competencies require competency in three areas (Exhibit 7.3):

1. Technical
2. Utility
3. Leadership (Kaminski, 2007)

In 2008 the NLN issued a statement with recommendations for schools of nursing to prepare students for practice in the dynamic health care arena. These recommendations are listed in Exhibit 7.4.

## Balancing Teaching, Scholarship, Service, and Institutional Demands

"True success as a faculty member is measured by the person's ability to juggle all aspects of the faculty role" (Finke, 2009, p. 6). The academic nurse educator's role usually includes three primary areas of responsibility:

- Teaching
- Scholarship
- Service

Some institutions, particularly those that have a practice-oriented focus, also include a fourth area, clinical service or practice. It is important to note that some institutions may put a higher emphasis on teaching but still expect academic faculty to meet certain criteria in the other areas.

## Use Feedback to Improve Role Effectiveness

Evaluation is another important responsibility of academic nurse educators. Not only can students provide valuable feedback to improve faculty effectiveness, faculty may also engage in self-evaluations and in the evaluation of their colleagues (Billings & Halstead, 2005). Peer evaluation is an important aspect of faculty development and is often included as part of the documentation required for promotion and tenure consideration.

The faculty evaluation process is complex and multifaceted and encompasses feedback regarding all areas of the faculty role. Sources of this important feedback include:

- Teaching evaluations from students, peers, and critiques/reviews of classroom teaching materials/activities.
- Reviews or critiques of scholarly works, such as:
    - Research (in progress or completed)
    - Grant proposals (submitted and/or funded)
    - Publications (journals, books, scholarly monographs, computer programs)
    - Presentations
- Feedback can be obtained regarding service on committees or participation in professional or community activities by requesting feedback from others.

| Exhibit 7.4 | NLN Recommendations for Preparing the Next Generation of Nurses to Practice in a Technology-Rich Environment |
|---|---|

*For Nursing Faculty*

■ Participate in faculty development programs to achieve competency in informatics.

■ Designate an informatics champion in every school of nursing to: (a) help faculty distinguish between using instructional technologies to teach vs. using informatics to guide, document, analyze, and inform nursing practice, and (b) translate state-of-the-art practices in technology and informatics that need to be integrated into the curriculum.

■ Incorporate informatics into the curriculum.

■ Incorporate ANA-recognized standard nursing language and terminology into content.

■ Identify clinical informatics exemplars, those drawn from clinical agencies and the community or from other nursing education programs, to serve as examples for the integration of informatics into the curriculum.

■ Achieve competency through participation in faculty development programs.

■ Partner with clinicians and informatics specialists at clinical agencies to help faculty and students develop competence in informatics.

■ Collaborate with clinical agencies to ensure that students have hands-on experience with informatics tools.

■ Collaborate with clinical agencies to demonstrate transformations in clinical practice produced by informatics.

■ Establish criteria to evaluate informatics goals for faculty.

*For Deans/Directors/Chairs*

■ Provide leadership in planning for necessary IT infrastructure that will ensure education that prepares graduates for 21st-century practice roles and responsibilities.

■ Allocate sufficient resources to support IT initiatives.

■ Ensure that all faculty members have competence in computer literacy, information literacy, and informatics.

■ Provide opportunities for faculty development in informatics.

■ Urge clinical agencies to provide hands-on informatics experiences for students.

■ Encourage nurse-managed clinics to incorporate clinical informatics exemplars that have transformed nursing practice to provide safe, quality care.

■ Advocate that all students graduate with up-to-date knowledge and skills in each of the three critical areas: computer literacy, information literacy, and informatics.

■ Establish criteria to evaluate outcomes related to achieving informatics goals.

*(Continued)*

| Exhibit 7.4 | NLN Recommendations for Preparing the Next Generation of Nurses to Practice in a Technology-Rich Environment (Continued) |
|---|---|

*For the National League for Nursing*

- Disseminate this position statement widely.
- Seek external funding and allocate internal resources to convene a think tank to reach a consensus on definitions of informatics, competencies for faculty and students, and program outcomes that include informatics.
- Participate actively in organizations that focus on education in nursing informatics to ensure that recommendations from those organizations are congruent with the NLN's positions on the curriculum.
- Use ETIMAC and its task groups to: (a) develop programs for faculty, showcasing exemplar programs, and (b) disseminate outcomes from the think tank.
- Encourage and facilitate accrediting bodies, regulatory agencies, and certifying bodies to reach a consensus on definitions related to informatics and minimal informatics competencies for practice in the 21st century.

From "Position Statement: Preparing the Next Generation of Nurses to Practice in a Technology-Rich Environment: An Informatics Agenda," by the National League for Nursing, May 9, 2008. *National League for Nursing.* Retrieved December 24, 2008, from http://www.nln.org/aboutnln/PositionStatements/informatics_052808.pdf

Faculty should seek out all relevant feedback related to their professional role. All data acquired should be utilized to design and individualize a plan to support continued growth and development in the faculty role.

## Engage in Self-Reflection for Professional Growth and Development

Academic nurse educators (as well as all nurses) have very specific accountabilities concerning lifelong learning (DeSilets & Dickerson, 2008; Yoder-Wise, 2008). Nurse educators should use reflection in a variety of circumstances as a means of maintaining professional competency including:

- Reflective teaching
- Reflective practice
- Reflective thinking (Bengtsson, 2003).

"A reflective assessment will help you realize accomplishments, assess new skills learned, and enable a learner to set new goals for future growth. A reflective assessment also allows the learner to reflect on personal feelings and reactions to a given situation" (Wagner, 2006, p. 30). This activity will provide the nurse educator with the opportunity to reflect on his or her career, educational needs, competencies, and future directions—all of which will have an impact on the pursuit of lifelong learning. One technique for conducting a comprehensive self-reflection is a 360-degree evaluation, a process of soliciting feedback about one's performance from multiple sources, including:

- Colleagues
- Students
- Administrators
- Subordinates

After collecting feedback, the nurse educator must analyze and reflect on the data collected and use this information to create a professional development plan. The benefits of this process, identified by Wagner (2006), include:

- "Reviewing data from sources other than just our own self-assessment will produce more accurate and valid pictures to our developed skills and abilities while illuminating the areas for continued growth" (p. 30).
- It "leads to an individual, specific, well-defined professional development plan" (p. 31).
- It improves one's ability to teach and, consequently, "influences the improvement of student achievement through the identification of truly authentic areas of strengths. When we are cognizant of our skill and knowledge strengths, we use them most efficiently" (p. 31).
- It "leads to innovative practices through the continuous process of setting and attaining goals" (p. 31).

It is important to keep in mind that reflection is a continuing process. As Collins et al. (2004) point out:

Reflective practice is key to ongoing professional growth and is identified as a critical component of professional development across a variety of fields. However, learning to be a reflective practitioner can be a challenging process. Growth comes from looking at your whole professional self instead of just the aspects with which you feel comfortable, [this is] a daunting and unfamiliar process for many (p. 144).

# CASE STUDIES

## Case Study 7.1

You are a new academic nurse educator, and next semester you are assigned to teach two sections of a medical surgical nursing course. One of the sections of the course will have traditional, four-year undergraduate nursing students, while the other section will have accelerated undergraduate nursing students. While planning the course and the use of technology, what types of technology could you use teaching this course? Would you use the same types of technology for both sections of the course? Would you use different types of technology for each section?

## Case Study 7.2

As part of your medical surgical nursing course you are asked to integrate a human simulation experience using standardized patients (patient actors). What type of simulation experience will you include? Will you include history taking, a physical exam, or patient teaching, or all three? What type of evaluation criteria will you include? Will the experience be a Pass/Fail experience, or will it have a specific grade? Who will evaluate the student? Who will do the debriefing session? Will you have the student do a self-evaluation or self-critique assignment?

## Practice Questions

1. An example of a Web 2.0 social networking site is
   A. Amazon
   B. eBay
   C. QVC
   D. Facebook

2. A standardized patient is
   A. A manikin that resembles a human
   B. A computerized manikin
   C. An actor who portrays a patient with a medical condition
   D. A computer program that simulates a patient scenario

3. Mentoring of nursing faculty includes which of the following
   A. Coaching
   B. Guiding
   C. Supporting
   D. All of the above

4. A comprehensive academic nurse educator orientation should include
   A. A review of available resources
   B. A review of administrative and governance structures
   C. An introduction to the culture and political environment
   D. All of the above

5. Which of the following describes a learner-directed activity
   A. A continuing education journal article
   B. An all-day Saturday live seminar
   C. A Webinar offered at a specific date and time
   D. A learning activity where the learner takes the initiative

6. The elements of lifelong learning for the nurse educator vary according to
   A. Career stages
   B. Type of faculty appointment

    C.  The mission of a university
    D.  All of the above

7.  A Wiki is
    A.  A collection of Web pages that are editable by anyone
    B.  A set of journal entries that are presented in reverse chronological order
    C.  A site designed to facilitate relationships and building strong connections/networks to strengthen a learning community
    D.  A method of distributing multimedia (audio or video) content (lectures, discussions, etc.) via the Internet for playback on mobile devices and personal computers

8.  The Technology Informatics Guiding Education Reform (TIGER) Initiative is
    A.  A government initiative to increase technology in education and health care
    B.  A non-profit specialty nursing organization
    C.  A consortium of more than 40 nursing professional organizations.
    D.  An HRSA initiative to increase technology skills in students and faculty

9.  Feedback during the faculty evaluation process can come from which of the following
    A.  Teaching evaluations
    B.  Peer evaluations
    C.  Critiques of scholarly work
    D.  All of the above

10.  Mentoring is
    A.  Eclectic and varied in its content and process
    B.  Involves reciprocal sharing, learning, and growth
    C.  Individually focused and takes time to evolve
    D.  All of the above

## References

ANA. (2000). *Scope and standards of practice for nursing professional development.* Washington, DC: Author.

ANCC. (2006). *Manual for accreditation of an approver or a provider of continuing nursing education.* Washington, DC: Author.

Bellack, J. P. (2004). Seasoned faculty: To retire or not? One solution to the faculty shortage—begin at the end. *Journal of Nursing Education, 43*(6), 243–244.

Billings, D. M., & Halstead, J. A. (2005). *Teaching in nursing: A guide for faculty* (2nd ed.). St. Louis, MO: Elsevier Saunders.

Bengtsson, J. (2003). Possibilities and limits of self reflection in the teaching profession. *Studies in Philosophy and Education, 22,* 295–316.

Brannan, J. D., White, A., & Bezanson, J. L. (2008). Simulator effects on cognitive skills and confidence levels. *Journal of Nursing Education, 47*(11), 495–500.

Brown, J. S. (2006). New learning environments for the 21st century. Author. Retrieved December 26, 2008, from http://www.johnseelybrown.com/newlearning.pdf

Collins, J. L., Cook-Cottone, C. P., Robinson, J. S., & Sullivan, R. R. (2004). Technology and new directions in professional development: Applications of digital video, peer review, and self-reflection. *Journal of Educational Technology Systems, 33*(2), 131–146.

DeSilets, L. D., & Dickerson, P. S. (2008). Recommendations for improving health care through lifelong learning. *The Journal of Continuing Education in Nursing, 39*(3), 100–101.

Finke, L. M. (2009). Teaching in nursing: The faculty role. In D. M. Billings & J. A. Halstead (Eds.), *Teaching in nursing: A guide for faculty* (pp. 1–68). St. Louis, MO: Elsevier.

Hasson, C., Cornelius, F., & Suplee, P. D. (2008). A technology driven nursing faculty resource center. *Nurse Educator, 23*(1), 22–25.

Kaminski, J. (2007). Nursing informatics competencies: Self-assessment. Author. Retrieved December 26, 2008, from http://www.nursing-informatics.com/niassess/index.html

National Education Association (NEA). (2007). NEA fact sheet. Author. Retrieved December 24, 2008, from http://www.nea.org/presscenter/neafact.html

National League for Nursing. (2001, September 19). Position statement: Lifelong learning for nursing faculty. *National League for Nursing* (p. 6). Retrieved December 24, 2008, from http://www.nln.org/aboutnln/PositionStatements/lifelong091901.pdf

National League for Nursing. (2005). Core competencies of nurse educators with task statements. *National League for Nursing.* Retrieved December 24, 2008, from http://www.nln.org/facultydevelopment/pdf/corecompetencies.pdf

National League for Nursing. (2006). Position statement: Mentoring of nurse faculty. *Nursing Education Perspectives, 27*(2), 110–113.

National League for Nursing. (2008, May 9). Position statement: Preparing the next generation of nurses to practice in a technology-rich environment: An informatics agenda. *National League for Nursing.* Retrieved December 24, 2008, from http://www.nln.org/aboutnln/PositionStatements/informatics_052808.pdf

Oermann, M. H. (2001). One-minute mentor. *Nursing Management, 32*(4), 12–13.

Saba, V. K., & McCormick, K. A. (2006). *Essentials of nursing informatics* (4th ed.). New York: McGraw-Hill.

Staib, S. (2003). Teaching and measuring critical thinking. *Journal of Nursing Education, 42*(11), 498–507.

Technology Informatics Guiding Education Reform (TIGER). (2007). The TIGER initiative: Evidence and informatics transforming nursing: 3-year action steps toward a 10-year vision. Retrieved December 26, 2008, from http://www.aacn.nche.edu/Education/pdf/TIGER.pdf

Wagner, K. (2006). Benefits of reflective practice. *Leadership, 36*(2), 30–32.

Wasburn, M. H. (2007). Mentoring women faculty: an instrumental case study of strategic collaboration. *Mentoring & Tutoring: Partnership in Learning, 15*(1), 57–72.

Yoder-Wise, P. S. (2008). Lifelong learning in nursing: A drilldown of the Macy foundation report. *The Journal of Continuing Education in Nursing, 39*(3), 99.

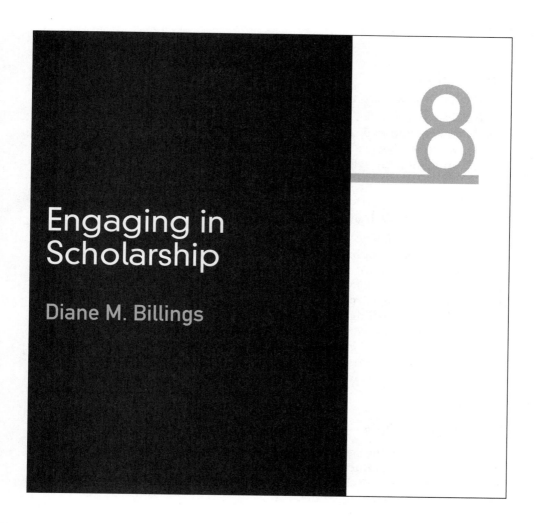

# Engaging in Scholarship

## Diane M. Billings

*Education is the most powerful weapon which you can use to change the world.*

—Nelson Mandela

**NLN Core Competency VII: Engage in Scholarship**

Nurse educators acknowledge that scholarship is an integral component of the faculty role, and that teaching itself is a scholarly activity (National League for Nursing [NLN], 2005, p. 22).

**Learning Outcomes**

- Discuss the meaning of scholarship in the nurse educator role.
- Identify the types of scholarship outlined by Boyer.
- Differentiate between the scholarship of teaching and the scholarship of teaching/learning.
- Identify attributes that comprise the science of nursing education.
- Appreciate the knowledge developed from evidence in education.

## Introduction

Being a scholar and engaging in scholarship is an important aspect of the role of the nurse educator. This chapter discusses the ways nurse educators can engage in scholarship and develop the science of nursing education. This chapter also discusses Boyer's model of scholarship and the Carnegie Foundation's work in promoting the scholarship of teaching and learning.

## Scholarship in Nursing Education

A *scholar* is a person who has particular knowledge in an area of specialization. A scholar has a spirit of inquiry and is able to think logically and communicate effectively. *Scholarship* is an inquiry process that results in outcomes, for example, innovations in teaching-learning strategies; the development of courses, course materials, and curricula; and the development of measures to assess and evaluate student learning. Scholarship in nursing education is recognized by peer reviews of the outcomes of teaching-learning practices, awards for teaching excellence, receipt of grants, and invitations to consult or share the scholarly work with others. Scholarship is also recognized by presentations, publications, and citation of the scholarly work by others.

## The Scholar's Role

The role of the nursing scholar is to develop and disseminate evidence for best practices in nursing education. The scholarly role is an expectation for nurse educators who work in schools of nursing situated in colleges and universities. The scholar's role is demonstrated by:

- Critiquing evidence for practice in nursing education
- Using evidence for teaching and learning practice
- Identifying issues for research
- Conducting research
- Disseminating findings
- Serving on committees of professional organizations
- Serving on editorial boards of journals related to teaching and learning

## Boyer's Model of Scholarship

Boyer's Model of Scholarship is one model that is used in many schools of nursing and institutions of higher learning to guide the work of faculty. The model, proposed by Ernest Boyer (1990), describes four types of scholarship that form the basis of scholarly work and contribute to effective teaching and learning. Although distinct in practice, the four types of scholarship are integrated. Boyer's four types of scholarship are:

- *Scholarship of discovery*: research or discovery of new knowledge; systematic inquiry; use of methods to develop a strong basis for practice-related knowledge.

*Example:* A nurse educator is using Podcasting with senior baccalaureate students. The nurse educator conducts a study to determine if the use of podcasting is appropriate for students with specific types of learning styles.

- *Scholarship of integration:* interpretation and synthesis of knowledge; may cross disciplinary boundaries.

*Example:* A nurse educator reviews the health sciences literature about using simulations for teaching students how to manage a diabetic crisis. She then uses the information to develop a multidisciplinary simulation for nursing students in an undergraduate nursing program.

- *Scholarship of application:* connects theory and practice; seeks to apply knowledge to significant problems; is translational work, assists end users to integrate the findings into their practices; application is also evident in service to the profession.

*Example:* A nurse educator who has an area of expertise in team-based learning presents the outcomes of the work at national meetings, and then consults with schools to help them integrate the method into their own academic programs and classrooms.

- *Scholarship of teaching:* The use of evidence to facilitate learning. The scholarship of teaching also involves identifying a problem, testing strategies, and making teaching and learning public through self-reflection, peer review, and the dissemination of work in appropriate disciplinary journals.

*Example:* A nurse educator developed a method of peer testing and has used the method in the classroom with outcomes of improved deep learning and higher test scores; students rate the method highly. The nurse educator develops a manuscript to share the findings of this approach to testing. The manuscript is accepted for publication for wider dissemination and potential further testing of the method in other classrooms. See Figure 8.1.

## 8.1   A model of Boyer's scholarship.

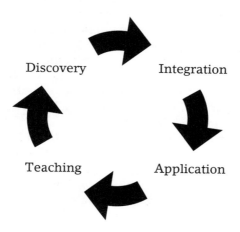

# Evidence-Based Education

Wieck (2003) affirms this in a study regarding the changes needed to attract the emerging workforce into nursing. She found that the top six traits the emerging workforce (i.e., the millennial generation) preferred were nursing faculty who were approachable, good communicators, professional, supportive, understanding, and motivating.

## The Use of Boyer's Model

Boyer's Model is used in nursing education as a framework for:

- Appointment
- Performance evaluation
- Promotion and tenure guidelines
- Organizing the professional portfolio

## Teaching, Scholarly Teaching, Scholarship of Teaching, and Scholarship of Teaching and Learning

Educators make a distinction among good teaching, scholarly teaching, the scholarship of teaching, and the Scholarship of Teaching and Learning.

- *Good teaching*
  Good teaching is typically defined by student satisfaction and positive student ratings of teaching (Allen & Field, 2005). Good teaching involves understanding the students and using effective teaching-learning practices.
- *Scholarly teaching*
  Scholarly teaching refers to nurse educators' use of practice wisdom, reflections on the effectiveness of one's own approach to teaching and evaluation, and the use of evidence to guide teaching practice (Allen & Field, 2005). Scholarly teaching involves a systematic study of teaching and learning practices and may result in the dissemination of knowledge through presentations and publications.
- *Scholarship of teaching*
  Scholarship of teaching refers to teaching that extends beyond the classroom (Allen & Field, 2005). Scholarship of teaching may include the development of products (simulations, books, games, and podcasts) that can be used by others. Scholarship of teaching also involves conducting research about teaching and learning.
- *The Scholarship of Teaching and Learning (SoTL)*
  The Scholarship of Teaching and Learning (SoTL) is an initiative of the Carnegie Foundation (Carnegie Academy for the Scholarship of Teaching and Learning, 2008) that builds on Boyer's Model of Scholarship to enhance the value of teaching, advocate for student learning, and bring

recognition to teaching as scholarly work. Many campuses have communities of faculty who collaborate to explore, share, and recognize each others' work to develop the scholarship of teaching and learning.

## The Science of Nursing Education

The science of nursing education refers to the research-based foundation on which the best practices for teaching nursing are developed and tested. Building the science of nursing education involves:

- Defining a significant problem
- Critiquing literature and identifying gaps
- Developing or using a framework to guide research
- Designing studies (classroom studies, multi-site studies, multi-method studies)
- Conducting studies
- Disseminating findings by sharing effective teaching or evaluation strategies and summaries of surveys about classroom practices. Dissemination also takes place when nurse educators present findings from research studies. Evidence of dissemination includes publications and presentations. Publications in peer reviewed and indexed journals are more highly valued than publications in journals with limited circulation or abstracts in conference proceedings and newsletters; the publication of scholarly work is preferred to presentations at scientific meetings.
- Using evidence in scholarship and research. The cycle of scholarship and research is complete when nurse educators base their curriculum development, teaching, evaluation, and use of technology on evidence. Evidence can be found in nursing journals which report study findings, at conferences where papers are presented, and at school and university scholarship days where the results of pilot studies and classroom research are presented. Increasingly, nursing education scholarship and research is interdisciplinary and evidence for nursing education practice is available in a variety of venues. All nurse educators must read the evidence, test it in their classrooms, and then determine the best practices for their own students.

## Evidence-Based Education

The advancement of nursing science requires nurse researchers to rethink the developmental phases of building research projects. Strategically forming, collaborating, and maintaining these alliances place nurse researchers in the position of leaders in research. This cross-disciplinary research is well suited for the complex health care issues experienced by patients, families, and communities (Loeb et al., 2008).

## Developing the Science of Nursing Education

Nurse educators also have responsibilities for developing the science of nursing education. Developing the science of nursing education:

> The NLNAC's model, "Pillars of Scholarship," incorporates Boyer's four scholarship categories (Stull & Lance, 2005).

- ■ Can be conducted by educators, regardless of educational preparation, who participate in the research process as leaders or members of a research team.
- ■ Requires the researcher and research team to maintain integrity as scholars by assuring the protection of human subjects, safeguarding data, using ethical approaches to inquiry, and collaborating with others.
- ■ Can involve collaboration with colleagues at the same and other institutions (multi-site research) and with colleagues in other disciplines (interdisciplinary research).

## Funding the Science of Nursing Education

Funding for nursing education research comes from a variety of sources. Professional nursing education organizations such as the NLN (Position Statement on Funding Nursing Education Research), National Nursing Staff Development Organization (NNSDO), American Association of College of Nursing (AACN), Sigma Theta Tau International, and a variety of specialty organizations have small grants programs to fund nursing education research. Also, most colleges and universities have small funds for classroom research.

## Evidence-Based Education

> McKenna, Bickle, and Caroll (2002), when examining Boyer's four stages of scholarship, identified a fifth stage, that of producing a scholarly product that is needed to meet tenure and promotion expectations. The authors share that "when teaching and research are perceived as two separate responsibilities, the passion for teaching may be diminished, and research may become a necessary burden" (p. 39). The key is to integrate the two.

## Evidence-Based Nursing Education

Evidence-based nursing education is the use of evidence to make decisions about developing educational programs, choosing the best teaching-learning strategies to achieve outcomes for a particular group of students in a particular setting, and selecting appropriate methods for evaluation. Evidence-based nursing education:

- ■ Draws on research in nursing education, higher education, psychology, and allied health disciplines

- Uses wisdom and accepted practices, and is guided by theory and empirical testing
- Questions existing teaching-learning practices that are unfounded, based in tradition, and have not been tested.

## Summary

Scholarship and producing scholarly work is one of the expectations of the role of the nurse educator. Boyer's Model describes four aspects of scholarship for guiding the appointment, retention, and promotion of nurse educators. Nurse educators both conduct research and develop the science of nursing education. Much more research is needed in nursing education to build a solid body of evidence and knowledge. Promoting the science of nursing education through evidence is imperative to guide our future in nursing. Without curriculum that is evidence-based and grounded in up-to-date science, the scholarship of education cannot survive. All four areas of Boyer's Model of Scholarship are intertwined; each is dependent on the others, as pictured in Figure 8.1.

# CASE STUDY

## Case Study 8.1

Three nurse educators team-teach a nursing skills course in a learning resources center, and each has responsibility for clinical supervision of 10 students on a medical-surgical nursing unit at the local hospital. One of the educators, an associate professor, has a PhD in clinical nursing; two of the nurses have MSN degrees in nursing and are clinical instructors. Scholarship is included in the appointment requirements for all faculty at the school of nursing.

The teaching team has noticed that students frequently break the sterile field when changing a sterile dressing. The nurse educators would like to conduct a study to determine if using simulation with a low-fidelity manikin vs. using return demonstration would improve the students' ability to change a sterile dressing correctly.

1. What is the evidence that needs to be obtained to determine the best practices for teaching students to change a sterile dressing?
2. What steps are needed to design the study?
3. What resources will the faculty need to conduct this study?
4. Will conducting the study fulfill requirements for producing "scholarly work" to meet the criteria for their rank?
5. What will be the most appropriate roles on the research team for each of these nurse educators?

## Practice Questions

1. A nurse educator is preparing a dossier for promotion to Associate Professor. The university uses Boyer's Model of Scholarship to guide the devel-

opment of the dossier. The nurse educator is providing evidence for the scholarship of application. The nurse educator should include which of the following examples to demonstrate excellence in the scholarship of application?

A. Funded research about the use of simulations to teach team collaboration.
B. Service on a task force of a national nursing organization in which the educator shares expertise about the use of rubrics for evaluating learning outcomes.
C. Published article in a highly rated peer-reviewed journal co-authored by an interdisciplinary team following the use of a case study to teach patient safety.
D. Receipt of a research award from a national nursing organization for establishing a program of research about problem-based learning.

2. The curriculum committee at a school of nursing is debating the best way to sequence clinical learning experiences. The committee should first
A. Contact other schools to see how they sequence their clinical courses.
B. Conduct a pilot test for one semester using three different approaches.
C. Review the published evidence.
D. Ask senior faculty about the sequence that has worked best in the past.

3. A nurse educator uses concept maps for the first time with nursing students in an accelerated program. The nurse educator is demonstrating which of the following?
A. Good teaching
B. Teaching excellence
C. Scholarship of teaching
D. Scholarly role

4. A nurse educator has completed a funded study about the effectiveness of the use of podcasts for nursing students with learning style preferences for auditory learning. Which of the following is the most effective way to share the results of this study?
A. Publish in a nursing education journal.
B. Present at national meeting of nurse educators.
C. Present at statewide meeting of educators in higher education.
D. Send the report of the findings to the funding agency.

5. Which of the following is the most effective form of peer review for scholarly work?
A. Written report from a department chair
B. Positive responses from colleagues on an online blog
C. Summary comments from a campus research support group
D. Grant funding from an agency external to the campus

6. A nurse educator wants to determine the effectiveness of using "debriefing" after a simulation in which students in her classroom interpreted an EKG and selected interventions for a critically ill "patient." In order to ob-

tain funding for this study, the nurse educator should first submit a proposal to
A.  American Association of Critical Care Nurses
B.  Campus small grants program for teaching innovations
C.  National League for Nursing
D.  Sigma Theta Tau International

*Brenda Reap-Thomson contributed the following questions.*

7.  The nurse educator analyzed data and reported outcomes of the safety regulations in an outpatient center. This would be an example of:
    A.  Scholarship of discovery
    B.  Scholarship of teaching
    C.  Scholarship of integration
    D.  Scholarship of practice (application)

8.  The students are encouraged to become members of the National Student Nurses' Association. The framework for this organization indicates that the students will gain experience:
    A.  Making decisions and being held accountable for those decisions
    B.  Following regulations determined by elected officers
    C.  Learning how to engage in social activities while in school
    D.  Discussing health information and presenting projects

9.  The university has received a grant to support the remedial education of minority students; this will provide assistance for more minorities' entrance into nursing. This would be an example of:
    A.  Research grants
    B.  Scholarship grants
    C.  Training grants
    D.  Program grants

10. A nurse educator is applying for a promotion. It would be of greatest advantage to
    A.  Write an article in a refereed journal
    B.  Write a chapter in a book
    C.  Present at a conference
    D.  Write an article for a non-refereed journal.

# References

Allen, M. N., & Field, P. A. (2005). Scholarly teaching and the scholarship of teaching: Noting the difference. *International Journal of Nursing Education Scholarship 2*(1). Retrieved November 13, 2008, from http://www.bepress.com/cgi/viewcontent.cgi?article=1094&context=ijnes

Boyer, E. (1990). *Scholarship reconsidered: Priorities of the professoriate.* San Francisco: Jossey-Bass.

Carnegie Academy for the Scholarship of Teaching and Learning. (2008). Retrieved November 25, 2008, from http://www.carnegiefoundation.org/programs/index.asp?key = 21

Loeb, S. J., Penrod, J., Kolanowski, A., Hupcey, J. E., Kopenhaver-Haidt, K., Fick, D. M., et al. (2008). Creating cross-disciplinary research alliances to advance nursing science. *Journal of Nursing Scholarship, 40*(2), 195–201.

McKenna, J., Bickle, M., & Carroll, J. B. (2002). Using scholarship to integrate teaching and research. *Journal of Family and Consumer Sciences, 94*(3), 39–45.

National League for Nurses (NLN). (2005). Core competencies for nurse educators with task statements. Retrieved May 1, 2009, from www.nln.org

Stull, A., & Lantz, C. (2005). An innovative model for nursing scholarship. *Journal of Nursing Education, 44*(11), 493–497.

Wieck, K. (2003). Faculty for the millennium: changes needed to attract the emerging workforce into nursing. *Journal of Nursing Education, 42*(4), 151–158.

# Functioning Effectively Within the Institutional Environment and Academic Community

## Mary Ellen Smith Glasgow

*To achieve all that is possible, we must attempt the impossible to be as much as we can be, we must dream of being more.*

—Gale Baker Stanton

### NLN Core Competency VIII: Function Within the Educational Environment

Nurse educators are knowledgeable about the educational environment within which they practice and recognize how political, institutional, social and economic forces impact their role (National League for Nursing [NLN], 2005, p. 23).

### Learning Outcomes

- Identify internal and external factors influencing nursing education.
- Describe the relationship of the mission of the parent institution to that of the nursing curriculum.
- Discuss the impact of an organizational climate on the development of the nurse educator.

■ Elaborate on the importance of a professional career development trajectory for nurse educators.

■ Investigate the concepts of mentorship and protégé as they relate to the educator role.

■ Analyze the nurse educator's leadership role with respect to institutional governance.

## Introduction

This chapter will focus on the nurse educator's roles and responsibilities within the institutional environment and academic community with particular emphasis on teaching, research/scholarship, and service requirements as well as internal and external forces affecting nursing education.

## Internal and External Forces Influencing Nursing and Higher Education

The faculty role in higher education has changed from that of a single-focused mission of teaching to a triad mission of teaching, scholarship, and service. Nursing education has changed dramatically from being housed in the service sector setting to the college and university setting (Finke, 2005). As nursing education entered the university setting, nursing faculty were held to the same research and scholarship standards as their non-nursing academic colleagues. The emphasis on research and scholarship continues to be a benchmark for nursing faculty productivity in university settings, particularly at research and comprehensive universities. There are many other internal and external forces influencing both nursing education and higher education today. These driving forces include:

■ Multiculturalism of society
■ Expanding technology, including distance education
■ Limited financial resources
■ Nursing faculty shortage
■ Nursing shortage
■ Aging population
■ Health disparities
■ Knowledge explosion
■ Emphasis on the "learner" instead of the "teacher" in relation to pedagogy
■ Increased demand for accountability
■ Outcomes assessment
■ Accreditation requirements
■ Federal funding
■ General economy
■ Political landscape

Enrollment, curriculum design, pedagogy, faculty expectations, faculty competencies, and scholarly productivity are all shaped by social, political, and economic forces. For example, societal multiculturalism will continue to shape curricula, and faculty will need to teach students to understand and respond effectively to the cultural and linguistic needs of patients they meet in health care encounters (Office of Minority Health, 2000). Today, changing demographics, culture, and linguistic diversity need to be emphasized in nursing curricula at all levels. Curricula need to be continually re-examined in light of these internal and external forces. It also is critical for nursing faculty to communicate nursing's value to the institution, academic community, and general public (Buresh & Gordon, 2006).

# Evidence-Based Education

Whitehead and Lacey-Haun (2004) report that nurses rank continuing nursing education as the third most vital component of nursing skill building. It is important to remember that many nurses are employed in settings without easy access to information about the evidence-based practices they are expected to use in patient care. A recent government report (Health Resources and Services Administration [HRSA], 2004) identified five major employment settings for nurses: hospitals (56%), community and public health settings (14.9%), ambulatory care settings (11%), nursing homes and extended care facilities (6.3%), and nursing education (2.6%). In addition, states are moving to mandating continuing nursing education as a requirement for license renewal (Yoder-Wise, 2008). As we move forward toward universal, state-mandated continuing nursing education, careful attention must be paid to the availability of and access to continuing nursing education information that is needed to fulfill this licensure requirement.

## Accreditation

- Halstead (2008) notes that two national professional nursing organizations currently accredit nursing education programs: the National League for Nursing Accrediting Committee (NLNAC) and the Commission for Collegiate Nursing Education (CCNE). The NLNAC accredits all nursing programs, including Licensed Practical Nursing, nursing diploma, Associate Degree, Baccalaureate Degree, Master's Degree, and Doctor of Nursing Practice (DNP) programs.

- The CCNE accredits Baccalaureate, Master's, and DNP degree programs.

- Research-focused doctoral programs (PhD, EdD, DNS, DNSc) and hybrid Clinical-Research Doctor of Nursing Practice Degree (DrNP, DNP) are not subject to accreditation. While post-Master's DNP programs are not required to be accredited, all BSN to DNP Programs that require new licensure (Certified Nurse Midwife, Nurse Practitioner, and Nurse Anesthetist) require accreditation.

- It must be noted that these are the current regulations; they are fluid and changing even as this book is being written.

- At present, CCNE will not accredit DNP programs that have an educator track as part of their core curriculum.

- Nursing education programs can choose to be accredited by either organization; some programs elect to be accredited by both organizations.
- The accreditation process provides an evaluative review of all components of the education program with an emphasis on program outcomes.
- Substantive components considered for accreditation include: curriculum, institutional and program governance, fiscal resources, instructional learning resources, student support services, faculty qualifications, student qualifications, faculty and student accomplishments, and a program evaluation plan that guides faculty program reviews and decision making.
- The process for both NLNAC and CCNE accreditation requires an on-site visit from faculty colleagues or peer reviewers from similar institutions.
- Prior to the on-site visit, faculty members prepare a written self-study report addressing each accreditation standard. It is important for faculty to have a clear understanding of the accreditation standards that guide the nature and execution of their nursing program.
- The NLNAC accreditation standards can be found online at http://www.nlnac.org/home.htm and CCNE accreditation standards can be found at www.aacn.nche.edu/Accreditation/index.htm.

## The Academic Setting

### College/University

- The organizational structures of American colleges and universities vary depending on institutional type, culture, and history, yet they also share much in common. While a private liberal arts and public research university in a state system may differ in terms of mission and focus, the vast majority of public and private universities are overseen by an institutional or system-wide governing board. Faculty self-governance is common in academia, and faculty members are involved in their campuses' strategic planning, fiscal oversight, curriculum planning, and student affairs.

### School of Nursing

- The school of nursing or nursing program's mission, philosophy, program outcomes, and curriculum are based on the college and university's mission.
- The expectations of the internal and external stakeholders need to be considered during program development or evaluation (Sauter & Applegate, 2005).

### Mission

- According to Csokasy (2005), a mission statement is a public statement of what an institution is about and why it exists.

- A mission statement provides direction for the planning of educational activities and provides clarity related to the target constituencies' goals of the institution related to teaching, research, and practice, and the level to which the institution aspires.
- The nursing educational mission is derived from the institution's mission statement, and the two mission statements need to be congruent with one another.
- The nursing educational mission statement describes the unique attributes of the program and provides direction for curriculum development.
- Curricular and structural changes need to consider the missions of both the university and its nursing program.

## Faculty Governance

- Finke (2005) describes how faculty have traditionally enjoyed the right of self-governance within the university setting.
- Self-governance includes developing policies related to student affairs, faculty expectations, faculty tenure and promotion guidelines, serving on faculty search committees, and developing, revising, and evaluating the curriculum.
- Faculty in partnership with academic administrators, who also hold a faculty rank in many instances, work collaboratively to address issues facing the university and larger academic community.

## Organizational Climate

- The organizational climate or culture is critical to the retention of nursing faculty, enthusiasm for innovation and learning, scholarly productivity, and clinical excellence.
- An organizational culture that encompasses the values and beliefs that the organization wants to promote is integral to any organization's success.
- The integration of values such as respect, collegiality, professionalism, and caring into the organizational culture fosters the development of its constituents.
- Leaders need to effect change, promote a positive organizational culture, articulate a vision, implement strategic plans, garner resources, network, and adapt to changing landscapes.
- The requisite leadership skills needed to oversee a program include aptitude, emotional intelligence, self-awareness, self-regulation, motivation, empathy, risk-taking, creativity, and social skills (Goleman, 2002; Grossman & Valiga, 2005).

## Collaboration, Partnerships, and Innovation

- In order to develop and maintain an innovative curriculum, nurse educators need to lead a cultural paradigm shift in nursing education that welcomes innovation, embraces creativity, and designs novel curricula and pedagogy that will ultimately improve the health and welfare of patients and professional nurses.

- Bellack (2005) challenges nurse leaders from within and across the public and private sectors to partner to "inspire and incite innovation and the transformation of nursing education."
- Strategic partnerships are one example of innovation as nurse leaders struggle to devise ways to manage the nursing shortage (Green et al., 2006).
- These strategic models of synergistic collaboration are being used to address issues of both nursing and nursing faculty shortages.
- Collaborative arrangements between academic and health care institutions allow partners to combine their respective strengths in achieving their mutual goals of increasing the registered nurse and nursing faculty workforce (Oermann, 2007; Puetz & Shinn, 2005).
- Typically, the Master's prepared nurse clinician is selected by the academic and health care institution to teach students in the clinical area based on his or her educational preparation, clinical expertise, and desire to teach, thus allowing the academic institution to increase its student enrollment (Tanner, 2005).
- Leaders need to create a safe, inclusive environment where faculty can feel comfortable regarding the adoption of innovative learning experiences.
- Visionary leaders are successful in developing partnerships in the organization while leading faculty and anticipating the effects of innovation by:
  - Staying focused on the educational program's core mission and values while being responsive to trends in the profession;
  - Identifying innovations of use to the institution; and
  - Encouraging faculty participation in planning changes with acceptable outcomes and having open discussions regarding the feasibility of the innovation in the institution (Murray, 2007).

## Evidence-Based Education

Interpersonal skills are important to the nursing role. Interpersonal skills can be assessed with the Conversational Skills Rating Scale (CSRS). It rates verbal and non-verbal behavior (Alexander, Vinzant, & McDaniel, 2008).

## Academic Responsibilities

### Teaching

- Elements of faculty participation in the teaching mission of an institution include (Finke, 2005):

- Effectiveness in undergraduate and graduate teaching in the class-room and/or clinical area
- Contributions to the curriculum, such as substantial revisions of existing courses, and the development of new courses and techniques for teaching
- Development of student evaluation methods
- Publications related to teaching, such as textbooks, manuals, articles, and so on.
- Effectiveness as an undergraduate and/or graduate adviser and/or mentor, including dissertation, thesis, or independent study advisement
- Teaching is evaluated based on student evaluations of teaching strategies, peer reviews of teaching strategies, evaluation of a teaching dossier, and assessment of student learning (Sauter & Applegate, 2005).

# Evidence-Based Practice

In a sample of more than 800 students enrolled in health-related programs at a large urban university, nursing students in the RN to BSN and graduate programs were found to be more field-dependent (cognitive style) than all other student groups, except for those in health information management programs. This put nursing students at a disadvantage in preparing for their profession. By using tailored educational strategies, nurse educators need to support field-dependent learners in didactic and clinical learning environments to ensure their success. Future research on selecting and the effectiveness of educational strategies, the use of technology, and the use of metacognition education (thinking about thinking) is needed for the field-dependent nursing student (Noble, Miller, & Heckman, 2008).

## Research/Scholarship

- Elements of faculty participation, particularly for tenure-track and tenured faculty, in a continuing program of research or other scholarship include:

  - Quantity and quality of research, or scholarship, as evidenced by publications, presentations of papers (including invited presentations nationally and internationally) and peer reviewed scholarship
  - Publications related to the advancement of pedagogical theory
  - Success in securing intramural (internal or institutional) funding
  - Success in securing extramural funding (external federal funding or private funding)
  - Effectiveness in directing the research of students
  - Originating, participating in, and/or directing research projects (Sauter & Applegate, 2005)

## Service

- Elements of faculty participation in service to the program, department, school or college, and university, and to the profession at the national and/or international level, include:

  - Leadership and/or participation in faculty elective bodies and service on committees at the program, department, college or school, and university levels
  - Faculty mentoring
  - Service to individual students and/or student organizations
  - Promotion of the university through extramural activities, such as recruitment events, alumni affairs, and so on
  - Other forms of service to the profession and society, such as serving on editorial boards, national organizations, and grant review panels (Finke, 2005)

# Appointment, Promotion, and Tenure

## Faculty Appointment

- Potential faculty candidates are invited to interview by a Faculty Search Committee appointed by a Dean or other university administrator. Faculty candidates may be asked to conduct a presentation about their research agenda or to demonstrate teaching competency during the interview process. Potential faculty candidates may also be interviewed by the department chair, Associate Dean for Research, and Dean, depending on the academic rank.
- Once considered for appointment, the faculty candidate's vita is reviewed by the appointment, promotion, and tenure committee, or another appropriate committee for the recommendation of faculty rank to the Dean. The academic ranks of Instructor, Assistant Professor, Associate Professor, and Professor are typically appointed based on the faculty candidate's teaching, research, and service experience and expertise.

## Academic Ranks

- Finke (2005) noted that appointment ranks, or tracks, have been developed to specify the responsibilities of faculty members in relation to teaching, scholarship, and service.
- Ranks include tenure, clinical, or research scientist. Clinical and research faculty have a prefix before their academic rank (e.g., Clinical Assistant Professor, or Research Associate Professor). Tenure-track and tenured faculty titles have no prefix.
- Tenure-track faculty are considered tenure-probationary until they achieve tenure. The tenure track is established for faculty whose primary responsibilities are teaching and research.

- The clinical faculty track has been developed at institutions for those faculty members whose primary responsibilities reside in clinical practice or the clinical supervision of students.
- The research scientist track is for faculty whose primary responsibilities are generating new knowledge and disseminating research findings.

## Non-Tenure Appointments

- Clinical and research faculty are generally non-tenured positions and are considered contracted faculty. Faculty members receive contracts on an annual or multi-year basis.

## The Appointment, Promotion, and Tenure Process

- The contemporary concept of tenure in U.S. colleges and universities can be traced to the "Statement of Principles of Academic Freedom and Tenure," which was adopted in 1940 by the American Association of University Professors and the Association of American Colleges, where the basic principles of tenure as a system to protect the academic freedom of faculty members were first articulated.
- Criteria for promotion and tenure are based on a university's overall mission and the Carnegie Foundation's university classification system; therefore, requirements vary among institutions.
- Promotion refers to advancement in rank. To be considered for promotion, faculty must submit a dossier as evidence of excellence in teaching, scholarship, and service.
- The criteria for tenure and/or promotion is established by the school/college and is evaluated by a committee of peers, school and university administrators, and the University Board of Trustees or other governing body.
- In most schools of nursing, a tenure track faculty member is appointed as an Assistant Professor and can expect to be promoted to the rank of Associate Professor at the time when tenure is granted.
- The American Association of University Professors (AAUP) can serve as a resource related to faculty rights pertaining to tenure and promotion. Their Web site is http://www.aaup.org/aaup.

# Career Development for Nurse Educators

Both new and experienced faculty need clear guidelines on career development and advancement in their respective academic institutions (Seldin, 2003).

## Developing a Career Trajectory

Successful faculty members have often developed a career development plan for themselves. Such a plan may include the following elements:

- Developing career goals

  - Short-term career goals
  - Long-term career goals

- Using effective time management

  - Identify the most productive intellectual time and protect it
  - Maximize value of scholarship and research time

- Understanding of the trajectory and stages of an academic career and the goals at each stage
- Mastery of negotiation and conflict resolution skills
- Developing a teaching portfolio
- Developing collaboration skills and the ability to maximize the benefits of collaboration while maintaining autonomy and boundaries
- Valuing the benefits of being mentored
- Developing a primary mentor-protégé relationship
- Consulting a coach to deal with any issues and barriers effectively (Doucette, 2008).

## Career Stages

Distinct behaviors are associated with various levels of faculty appointments. These can generally be described for each faculty level as noted below.

- Instructor

  - Develop skills in the scholarship of discovery (research or discovery of new knowledge)
  - Develop skills in the scholarship of teaching
  - Develop skills in scholarship of integration (interpretation and synthesis of knowledge across discipline boundaries in a manner that provides new insights)
  - Develop skills in the scholarship of application of knowledge (connects theory and practice) (Boyer, 1997)
  - Understand the responsibilities of protégé and mentor

- Assistant Professor

  - Develop an area of expertise
  - Pose and address an important question or focus in that area that has the potential for significant findings or impact (scholarship or research)
  - Develop oneself autonomously within this area
  - Develop one's own laboratory for evaluating these questions, whether the lab is a wet-bench laboratory, the skills, staff, and resources for clinical, population-based or teaching investigation, or another setting (i.e., demonstrating the ability to function scientifically as an "independent" investigator)
  - Lead or collaborate in the development and evaluation of an innovative educational program

- Present findings from this work at appropriate national meetings and/or publish the results of this work in peer-reviewed journals
- Obtain external, peer-reviewed funding to support this work
- Become nationally recognized for this body of work, whether it be clinical research or education
- Initiate or continue to compile the teaching portfolio (Seldin & Miller, 2008)
- Provide faculty teaching and service to the nursing department

- Associate Professor

  - Continue research/scholarship in one's area of expertise as an autonomous investigator and in publication productivity
  - Become an interdependent investigator and/or leader
  - Continue with the activity of developing and evaluating innovative educational programs
  - Establish a body of contributions that one can make in one's defined area; become nationally and internationally recognized for this work
  - Take on responsibility for an area important to one's own institution, becoming a resource and leader recognized beyond one's department
  - Mentor junior faculty in a productive manner
  - Demonstrate peer-reviewed awards, honors, or other indications of excellence
  - Demonstrate peer-reviewed support for research or program development
  - Become involved at the national level through involvement in societies reflective of one's expertise
  - Serve on national committees such as study sections
  - Serve on departmental and university functions, particularly some time-consuming committees

- Professor

  - Continue to demonstrate leadership in research, teaching, and service
  - Function as a role model
  - Enhance the mentoring role and, in particular, assist junior faculty in their career development

## Choosing a Mentor

- A faculty mentor either can be assigned to the protégé, or the mentor and protégé can mutually agree upon the relationship. The mentoring relationship is generally consultative and constructive in most institutions; however, some schools have a more prescriptive approach (Sauter & Applegate, 2005).
- Grossman and Valiga (2005) define a mentor as an individual who assists his or her protégé as he or she works to establish a professional

reputation. The mentor provides support and guidance during times of stress while assisting in the development and enhancement of the protégé's professional skills.

■ The mentor helps the protégé learn the political landscape, expand his or her network, gain professional insight, and foster personal and professional growth.

■ An authentic mentor invests a great deal of time and effort into the advancement of his or her protégé. The mentor-protégé relationship is conscious, purposeful, and typically lasts for a number of years.

■ A mentor looks for the following attributes in the protégé:

    ■ Intelligence
    ■ Strong work ethic
    ■ Initiative
    ■ Integrity
    ■ Professional demeanor
    ■ Commitment
    ■ Ability to accept feedback
    ■ Intellectual curiosity

■ A protégé looks for the following attributes in the mentor:

    ■ Intelligence
    ■ Someone who is willing to invest in him or her
    ■ Willingness to give feedback
    ■ Strong networking capabilities
    ■ Professional contacts
    ■ Ability to motivate
    ■ Integrity

## Faculty Development

■ According to Donnelly (2008), for new nurse educators, a substantive, formal orientation to the nursing program and institution is essential. During this orientation, new faculty members begin the process of socialization into the academy. A faculty orientation program is particularly critical for novice faculty who need to understand the expectations for tenure and promotion and the sociopolitical issues of the institution (Sauter & Applegate, 2005).

> Any program that ignores the sociopolitical forces in the external environment will do a disservice to its graduates (Bowen, Lyons, & Young, 2000).

    ■ Nurse educators need to understand the mission and goals of the institution, nature of the curriculum, academic policies and procedures, the organization of the program, the school and how it fits into the university, and the structure and charges of the various nursing and university committees.

- Seasoned nurse educators should be involved in these orientation and development sessions to facilitate collegial relationships, impart knowledge and expertise, and to encourage mentor-protégé relationships.
- The use of travel monies to attend conferences, seminars, and research colloquia are critical to faculty development.
- Finke (2005) stated that ongoing support and professional development is needed for nurse educators throughout their careers in the following areas:

  - Curriculum development, teaching, using teaching, learning, and information resources, and evaluating student outcomes
  - Professional practice
  - Relationships with students and colleagues
  - Service and faculty governance
  - Scholarship
  - Mentoring

## The Curriculum Vita and Professional Portfolio/Dossier

- A curriculum vita—often called a CV or vita—is used for academic positions. Thus, vitae tend to provide great detail about academic and research experiences. While resumes tend toward brevity, vitae lean toward completeness (Seldin, 2003). A sample curriculum vita format can be found in Exhibit 9.1.
- The professional portfolio/dossier is typically used to display one's work when applying for appointments, promotions, and tenure. A portfolio or dossier should include sample publications, syllabi, teaching evaluations, and recommendation letters. A portfolio or dossier is a practical way to reflect upon and document one's teaching, research, and service (Seldin, 2003; Seldin & Associates, 2006; Seldin & Miller, 2008).

  - In recent years, electronic portfolios have come into use in academic institutions as a means for students to display their work and demonstrate competency related to writing, clinical objectives, and so on.

# CASE STUDY

## Case Study 9.1

A new doctorally prepared faculty member has just completed her faculty orientation at the school of nursing. You have been assigned as her mentor. What questions would you want to ask this new faculty member regarding her career trajectory plan? As her mentor, what is important to convey to the faculty member given her career stage?

| Exhibit 9.1 | Sample Curriculum Vita |
| --- | --- |

A curriculum vitae should include the following items:

1. Name in full
2. Current home and mailing address, telephone number, fax number, and e-mail address
3. Education
   A. List of degrees, with the last degree listed first
   B. For each degree, include name of college/university, year degree granted, major(s)/concentration(s), minor(s), title of dissertation/thesis, if applicable
   C. Postgraduate training
      i. List chronologically, starting with most recent position
      ii. Give years, institutions, and type of training
4. Employment history
   A. List chronologically, starting with the most recent position held and including consulting positions, if applicable
   B. Indicate each place of employment and years employed
5. Certification and licensure (including recertification)
6. Military service
7. Honors and awards
   A. Starting with the most recent, list chronologically by name of the award
   B. Include each awarding institution and/or organization
   C. Indicate the nature of each award if not apparent
8. Memberships and offices in professional societies
9. Professional committees and administrative service
   A. Institutional: Committees on which you have served or chaired, including years of membership
   B. Extramural (local, regional, national, international). Include the following:
      i. Membership on editorial boards
      ii. Editorship of symposia volumes, texts, or journals
      iii. Service as an examiner for a professional organization
      iv. Reviewer of grants for extramural funding sources
      v. Reviewer of manuscripts for journal publications
      vi. Convener of symposia, conferences, or workshop in one's field and/or profession
   C. Name of each organization or publication, your role, and years of service
10. Community service (service not related to the institution but provided by you, either in your profession or in some other capacity)
    A. List chronologically, earliest first
    B. Give your role and the organization
11. Educational activities
    A. Courses/Clerkships/Programs
       i. Taught
       ii. Coordinated
       iii. Developed

*(Continued)*

Exhibit
9.1    Sample Curriculum Vita (Continued)

    B. Advising/Mentoring/Tutoring: For each of the above categories include course title, audience, and years of involvement

    C. Educational Materials: List texts, atlases, CAI, manuals, evaluation tools, etc., developed that were used only within the institution

12. Clinical activities

    A. Outline of major clinical activities including the following:

        i. Rounds, clinics

        ii. Development and/or implementation of clinical programs, quality assessment of programs

    B. Health care education in the lay community

        i. Presentations

        ii. Publications in the lay press

13. Support

    A. List past and present extramural support received

    B. List past and present intramural support received. Include role in the project, title of study, funding agencies, including appropriate ID number, effective dates, and total amount of award

    C. List grant applications already submitted and still pending, with the same information as above

14. Graduate students, postdoctoral fellows, and postgraduate trainees

    A. List the graduate students who have received advanced degrees (Master's, PhD) with you as their supervisor. Give the name of each student and years of study, thesis title, date when degree was awarded, program/department in which study was done, and institution awarding degree

    B. List postdoctoral fellows and postgraduate trainees and visiting scientists who have been under your direct supervision for their training. Give names, years, research or clinical study, and means of support (if training grant or NRSA)

15. Bibliography

To be listed under the following separate headings and according to APA (American Psychological Association) style. N.B.: items "accepted for publication" and/or "submitted for publication" should be so indicated and should include, together with the following information, the expected date of publication and/or date of submission

A. Published full-length papers

    1. Provide a chronological list with complete citations, including the following:

        i. Names and initials of all authors

        ii. Titles of the articles

        iii. Name of journal, volume, page numbers, year

    2. Indicate if peer-reviewed by using an asterisk before the citation

B. Books and chapters in books including page numbers. Provide complete citations, including press and city of printing

C. Communications, such as videotapes, discs, slide atlases, computer programs, etc., used by others outside the institution

*(Continued)*

| Exhibit 9.1 | Sample Curriculum Vita (Continued) |
| --- | --- |

D. Book reviews, letters to editors (when these are not articles, which they can be, as in *Nature* [London] or *J. Mol. Biol.*). Provide complete citations.

E. Abstracts (optional, but if included, provide complete citations). Indicate by asterisk if peer reviewed

16. Presentations

A. By invitation: May include invited seminar presentations (except those for job interviews) and presentations at conferences, society meetings, professional boards

B. By competition or peer-review

For each presentation, provide type, full title, date and place presented, and the auspices presented under (program, department, college, university, society, etc.) Use, wherever possible, the APA style.

## Practice Questions

*Contributed by Brenda Reap Thompson.*

1. A nurse educator is discussing graduation with students. One of the students says that being responsible for clients without the presence of an instructor is very frightening. Which statement by the nurse educator would be most appropriate?
   A. "The nurse manger will be available to guide you in decision making related to client care."
   B. "Most hospitals have an orientation program that will make sure you are prepared."
   C. "The Procedure Manual is always available to assist you in making client care decisions."
   D. "Your mentor will provide a structured process to guide your decisions and behaviors."

2. The school of nursing has implemented a standardized examination to be administered at the mid-curriculum completion point. What is the purpose of the examination? Select all that apply.
   A. Identify students who are below the benchmark.
   B. Determine if there is a need to revise the curriculum.
   C. Provide another method of testing to add to students' grades.
   D. Collect data that can be used for informational purposes.

3. A nurse educator is mentoring a new educator. The new educator looks stressed and says, "I had some problems with the class, but I know things will get better." Which of the following responses would be appropriate?
   A. "Tell me about your class."
   B. "Do you want to meet sometime to discuss your problem?"

    C.  "It takes a few weeks to get used to the students."

    D.  "Do you need me to help you?"

4.  A nurse educator is teaching a large class that is very diverse. Which population of students is at increased risk for failure?

    A.  Students who decided to pursue a second career.

    B.  Students who just graduated from high school.

    C.  Students who speak English as a Second Language (ESL).

    D.  Students who transferred from another program in the college.

5.  A nurse educator has a student in class who receives accommodations for increased time for testing because of a disability. The faculty needs to:

    A.  Understand the nature of the disability.

    B.  Meet privately with the student.

    C.  Accommodate the student.

    D.  Keep a copy of the letter from the physician.

6.  A student who was unsuccessful in the course tells a faculty member that she does not think it was her fault she failed. She said that she came to every class, but that the tests were unfair. Which of the following statements by the faculty would be appropriate?

    A.  "You can appeal the grade if you think it was unfair."

    B.  "Only four students out of sixty failed the course."

    C.  "How many hours per week did you spend studying?"

    D.  "Are your grades better in your other courses?"

7.  The chair of the Curriculum Committee is known as a transformational leader. This indicates that the leader:

    A.  Developed within the committee to accomplish a task.

    B.  Provided opportunities for the committee to make choices.

    C.  Acted quickly to complete the objectives of the committee.

    D.  Energized the committee to perform at a high level.

8.  A clinical instructor provided learning opportunities for four students. Which of the following clinical experiences reflects use of the affective domain?

    A.  Taking vital signs on a client who is receiving a blood transfusion.

    B.  Demonstrating tracheal suctioning of a client with asthma.

    C.  Interviewing a client who was diagnosed last week with breast cancer.

    D.  Developing a care plan for a client with Type I Diabetes Mellitus.

9.  A faculty member is completing a peer review. During the adult health class, the students sit quietly; some learners take notes, and some just listen to the lecture. Which of the following information would be appropriate to suggest?

    A.  Pause frequently during the lecture to ask students if they have questions.

    B.  Initiate a game that involves all students in a quick review of the content.

    C.  Add pictures of anatomical structures to the PowerPoint lecture to promote student understanding.

    D.  Give an unannounced quiz to determine if students understand the content that was taught.

10. The course data demonstrates that 97% of the class passed the course. The class average on the customized specialty external examination, which is 15% of the grade, was 70.5%. Which conclusion can be drawn from this data?
    A. The internal curriculum evaluation should be reviewed.
    B. The students studied harder for the internal examinations.
    C. The class was unable to complete all of the objectives of the course.
    D. The students are less familiar with computerized examinations.

11. A nurse educator taught cardiac rhythms, code management and medications in the Adult Critical Care Course. What would be the *most* effective method of determining the students' understanding of the information?
    A. Ask students to write a one minute paper about what they learned in class today.
    B. Provide a case study and let the students answer the questions as a group.
    C. Schedule a simulation experience that will encompass the chapter objectives.
    D. Include five questions for each hour of teaching in the unit examination.

# References

Alexander, J., Vinzant, J., & McDaniel G. S. (2008, September 19). *Assessing interpersonal skills.* Paper presented at the NLN Educational Summit, San Antonio, TX.

Bellack, J. (2005, April). *Health professions education: The demands of the new environment.* Paper presented at the meeting of the Robert Wood Johnson Executive Nurse Fellows Program Leadership Seminar, Chicago, IL.

Bowen, M., Lyons, K. J., & Young, B. E. (2000). Nursing and health care reform: Implications for curriculum development. *Journal of Nursing Education, 39*(1), 27–33.

Boyer, E. L. (1997). *Scholarship reconsidered: Priorities of the professoriate.* New York: Jossey-Bass.

Buresh, B., & Gordon, S. (2006). *From Silence to Voice: What Nurses Know and Must Communicate to the Public* (2nd ed.). New York: Cornell University Press.

Csokasy, J. (2005). Philosophical foundations of the curriculum. In D. Billings & J. Halstead (Eds.), *Teaching in nursing: A guide for faculty* (pp. 125–144). St. Louis, MO: Elsevier.

Donnelly, G. (2008). Faculty retention. In H. Feldman (Ed.), *Nursing leadership: A concise encyclopedia* (pp. 214–216). New York: Springer Publishing.

Doucette, J. N. (2008). Coaching nurses. In H. Feldman (Ed.), *Nursing leadership: A concise encyclopedia* (pp. 114–115). New York: Springer Publishing.

Finke, L. M. (2005). Teaching in nursing: The faculty role. In D. Billings & J. Halstead (Eds.), *Teaching in Nursing: A Guide for Faculty* (pp. 3–20). St. Louis, MO: Elsevier.

Goleman, D. (2002). *Primal leadership.* Boston: Harvard Business School Press.

Green, A., Fowler, C., Sportsman, S., Cottenoir, M., Light, K., & Schumann, R. (2006). Innovation in Nursing Education: A Statewide Grant Initiative. *Policy, Politics, & Nursing Practice, 7*(1), 45–53.

Grossman, S. C., & Valiga, T. M. (2005). *The new leadership challenge: Creating the future of nursing.* Philadelphia: F.A. Davis Company.

Halstead, J. A. (2008). Accreditation in nursing education. In H. Feldman (Ed.), *Nursing leadership: A concise encyclopedia.* New York: Springer Publishing.

Health Resources and Services Administration (HRSA). (2004). *The registered nurse population: Findings from the 2004 National Sample Survey of Registered Nurses.* Retrieved April 2, 2009, from http://bhpr.hrsa.gov/healthworkforce/rnsurvey04/3.htm

Murray, T. A. (2007). Innovation in nursing education: Which trends should you adopt? *Nurse Educator, 32*(4), 154–160.

National League for Nurses (NLN). (2005). Core competencies for nurse educators with task statements. Retrieved May 1, 2009, from www.nln.org

Noble, K. A., Miller, S. M., & Heckman, J. (2008). The cognitive style of nursing students: Educational implications for teaching and learning. *Journal of Nursing Education, 47*(6), 245–253.

Oermann, M. H. (2007). *Annual review of nursing education, Volume 6: Clinical nursing education.* New York: Springer Publishing.

Office of Minority Health. (2000). *Assuring cultural competence in health care: Recommendations for national standards and an outcomes-focused research agenda.* Retrieved November 13, 2008, from http://www.omhrc.gov/clas/finalpo.htm

Puetz, B., & Shinn, L. (2005). Strategic partnerships. *Journal of Nursing Administration, 32,* 182–184.

Sauter, M. K., & Applegate, M. H. (2005). Educational Program Evaluation. In D. Billings & J. Halstead (Eds.), *Teaching in nursing: A guide for faculty* (pp. 543–599). St. Louis, MO: Elsevier.

Seldin, P. (2003). *The teaching portfolio: A practical guide to improved performance and promotion/tenure decisions* (3rd ed.). Boston: Anker Publishing Co.

Seldin, P., & Associates. (2006). *Evaluating faculty performance: A practical guide to assessing teaching, research, and service.* Boston: Anker Publishing Co.

Seldin, P., & Miller, E. J. (2008). *The academic portfolio: A practical guide to documenting teaching, research, and service.* San Francisco: Jossey-Bass.

Tanner, C. A. (2005). What are our priorities? Addressing the looming shortage of nurse faculty. *Journal of Nursing Education, 44,* 247–248.

Whitehead, T. D., & Lacey-Haun, L. (2004). Evolution of accreditation of continuing nursing education in America. *The Journal of Continuing Education in Nursing, 39*(11), 493–499.

Yoder-Wise, P. S. (2008). Thank you to our peers. *Journal of Continuing Education in Nursing, 39*(11), 484.

# Comprehensive Practice Questions

*Mary Gallagher-Gordon, Brenda Reap Thompson, Dr. Frances Cornelius, Dr. Ruth Wittmann-Price, Dr. Marylou McHugh, and Dr. Rosemary Fliszar, and Maryann Godshall contributed these questions.*

1. The following statistics were calculated on a multiple-choice question on an exam:

   | Point Biserial = 0.61 | Correct answer = C | | Total group = 76.47% | |
   |---|---|---|---|---|
   | Distractor Analysis: | A | B | C | D |
   | Pt-Biser.: | −0.59 | 0.00 | 0.61 | −0.24 |
   | Frequency: | 6% | 0% | 88% | 6% |

   The reason for this frequency distribution for distractor B is:

   A. students who scored higher on the exam got the answer wrong
   B. the distractor was not clear
   C. this distractor has been used on previous exams
   D. this distractor is too easy

   *Correct answer is D: Distractor B needs to be replaced because it did not differentiate.*

2. An educator is reviewing the item analysis for the final examination. Which conclusion would be accurate for this correct item on the examination?

   N = 100
   P = 0.71
   Correct Answer = C

   | Options | A | B | C | D |
   |---|---|---|---|---|
   | N | 12 | 11 | 70 | 7 |
   | Pt Biserial | −0.12 | −0.26 | +0.29 | +0.06 |

   A. The item is too difficult for this level of students and should be revised.
   B. The item tested well and should be utilized for future testing in this course.
   C. Option D may also be correct, since the higher-level students chose that answer.
   D. Option A should be changed, since a large percentage of students chose that answer.

*The correct answer is B. The P value = 0.71, which indicates that the question was somewhat challenging for students, as 0.90 indicates an easy item and 0.30 indicates the most difficult item.*

*The Pt Biserial 0.20–0.29 indicates a good item; 0.30–0.39 indicates an excellent item.*

*The item is a higher level item and was challenging for many students.*

*C. Answer D was chosen by students with a positive Pt Biserial, but the higher-level students chose the correct answer.*

*D. The students who chose option A had a negative Pt Biserial, which means they scored lower on the examination.*

3. The educator reviews the item analysis for the pediatric examination. Which conclusion would be accurate for this item on the examination?

N = 100
P = 0.45
Correct Answer = A

| Options | A | B | C | D |
|---|---|---|---|---|
| N | 68 | 4 | 8 | 20 |
| Pt Biserial | 0.06 | −0.06 | −0.09 | 0.19 |

   A. The higher-level students got the item incorrect, so the question should be reviewed.
   B. Most of the class got the item correct, so there are no necessary revisions needed at this time.
   C. Option B should be revised, since a small percentage of the class chose that answer.
   D. Option D is a good distracter, since one-fifth of the class chose that answer.

*The correct answer is A. The P value = 0.45, indicating that the question was very challenging for students, since 0.90 indicates an easy item and 0.30 indicates the most difficult item.*

*The Pt Biserial below 0.10 should be reviewed, since 0.10–0.14 indicates a marginal item.*

*Even though most of the class got the item correct, the Pt Biserial for the correct answer showed the item did not test well.*

*C. Option B does not need revisions.*

*D. Option D had a positive Pt Biserial which was higher than the key. Students who chose this option were higher-level students. The Pt Biserial should not be higher than the key.*

4. The nurse educator at the clinical site is co-signing client care notes provided by a student. The educator's signature attests that:

   A. The client received the wound dressing care exactly as stated in the documentation.
   B. The student reported the dressing on the client's right leg was changed.

C. The instructor observed the student completing the wound dressing.

D. The client's wound dressing has today's date noted on the tape.

*The correct answer is A. The nurse educator's signature verifies that the care was provided and that the information on the chart is accurate.*

*B, C, and D are incorrect.*

5. A nurse educator has eight students on a medical-surgical floor. Which situation may indicate that the nurse educator is at risk for negligence?

A. The client was walking to the bathroom with the assistance of the student; the client fell and fractured the right femur.

B. The client developed hives after an antibiotic was administered by the student; the nurse added the allergy to the client's data.

C. The client returned from surgery and developed shock from hemorrhage; the student had been monitoring the client's vital signs.

D. The client's 8:00 A.M. medications were not administered because the gastrostomy tube was obstructed; the student reported it to the nurse.

*The correct answer is C. The faculty member could be liable because of a breach of responsibilities, such as lack of student supervision or inappropriate client assignment. The student was monitoring vital signs of a client who had just returned from surgery; therefore, the client was unstable. Students cannot be expected to recognize early clinical manifestations of complications.*

*A. Students can be sued and are responsible for their own conduct when providing client care. The nurse educator would not need to be present during the ambulation of a client.*

*B. The client did not have a documented allergy to the medication on the chart; therefore, this would not be an indication of negligence.*

*D. The student demonstrated accountability by notifying the nurse. Medications could be prescribed to be administered by another route. This would not be an indication of negligence.*

6. Class was cancelled because of extreme weather conditions; there are only two weeks left in the semester. Which of the following assignments would be the most appropriate method for completing the course work?

A. Instructing students to outline the chapter focusing on key points.

B. Encouraging students to answer the questions at the end of the chapter.

C. Informing students to respond to the case study posted to the class' Blackboard discussion.

D. Telling students to bring any questions about content to the next class.

*The correct answer is C. Case studies promote critical thinking. Responding to information posted by their colleagues on Blackboard allows students to be interactive. Faculty can also determine if all students responded.*

*A. D will promote learning, however there is no critical thinking involved in the assignment.*

*B. The questions may promote critical thinking, but it provides no interaction with other students.*

7. An example of a political organization that may be instrumental in helping advance nursing's agenda is:

    A. ANA
    B. OSHA
    C. ACLU
    D. HL7

    *The correct answer is C. The American Civil Liberties Union (ACLU) is an excellent organization for partnering with nursing and advancing agendas.*

8. A nurse educator is working on a leadership committee to craft a school mission statement. Which leadership competency is the nurse demonstrating?

    A. Conceptual
    B. Technical
    C. Governance
    D. Political

    *The correct answer is C. A mission statement is one of the governance pieces of the program.*

9. During the immediate aftermath of Hurricane Katrina, a nurse establishes a triage center at a local elementary school. Using the school as a base, the nurse organizes a group of volunteers to go door-to-door in the community to locate people who need care. This is an example of which leadership theory:

    A. Innovation
    B. Trait
    C. Great Events
    D. Transformational Leadership

    *The correct answer is C. It is a great event or crisis situation to which this leader has responded.*

10. A nurse educator works with an interdisciplinary team consisting of nurses, computer engineers, and programmers on a committee charged with the task of creating an innovative mobile decision support application. The nurse provides guidance regarding technical design specifications and output expectations. This demonstrates the integrative element of:

    A. Idea generation
    B. Idea structuring
    C. Idea dissemination
    D. Idea promotion

    *The correct answer is C. Idea structuring is used to frame the project in terms of functionality and usability.*

11. A nurse educator is charged with the task of evaluating a school's effectiveness following a transformative organizational change and restructuring that occurred in response to some major economic influences. The nurse educator understands that the evaluation model most appropriate in this instance would likely be:

A. Total quality management model
B. Satisfaction model
C. Resource-input model
D. Organizational learning model

*The correct answer is D. The organization learning model will evaluate if the system responded effectively to change.*

12. Change can be driven by many sources of influence. Incentives, such as increased pay or promotions, are sources of influence drawn from:

A. Personal ability
B. Social motivation
C. Structural motivation
D. Structural ability

*The correct answer is C. Structural motivators are those built into the system itself, such as pay raises or promotions.*

13. According to Berwick, the rate at which a change occurs is linked to the presence of certain elements. Change is likely to occur faster if the following is present:

A. Ability to "reinvent" the innovation
B. Decision-makers understand the innovation
C. Consensus among stakeholders
D. Entrepreneurial spirit within the organization

*The correct answer is A. Reinventing the innovation refers to the notion of keeping an idea alive in a system.*

14. Roger's identifies five steps in the process of diffusion of innovation. The third step is:

A. Knowledge: The decision-making unit begins to understand the innovation.
B. Implementation: The innovation is put to use.
C. Decision: Activities lead to a decision to adopt or reject the innovation.
D. Confirmation: The individual or decision-making unit seeks reinforcement that the decision was correct.

*The correct answer is C. The third step is the decisional stage, wherein actors decide if the structure will adopt the change.*

15. According to Berwick, the rate at which a change occurs is linked to: (select all that apply)

    A. Perceptions of the innovation/change
    B. Characteristics of the people who adopt the innovation
    C. Contextual factors associated with the organization
    D. Leadership style within the organization

    *The correct answers are A, B, and C. All answers but D are a predictor of change. Individual leadership should not be predictive of change.*

16. Which of the following statements related to Roger's Diffusion of Innovation theory is correct?

    A. It is always spontaneous and unplanned
    B. It includes a pre-contemplation phase
    C. A person's motivation is a central concept
    D. It is communicated through channels

    *The correct answer is D. Roger's diffusion theory is always communicated through channels, as opposed to unstructured or spontaneous communication.*

17. A discussion erupts at a nurse educator seminar about students failing and the various progression policies of each school. One of the participants states that she does not like some of her school's progression policies because she feels they are injurious to the students' dignity. You would suspect her teaching philosophy to be?

    A. Emancipatory
    B. Humanism
    C. Behaviorism
    D. Constructivism

    *The correct answer is B. Humanism holds the protection of human dignity as its primary goal.*

18. A nurse educator is assessing another nurse educator's teaching style. Which information is most important for the nurse educator to obtain?

    A. The assignments he or she gives the class
    B. His or her relationship with the students
    C. The teaching strategies he or she uses in the classroom
    D. The patients he or she assigns the students in clinical situations

    *The correct answer is B. One's teaching style is related to the manner in which the educator relates (or does not relate) to the learners.*

19. It is important to assess a new nurse educator's knowledge of critical thinking strategies because one of the best ways to facilitate students' critical thinking is to?

    A. Role model behaviors for students
    B. Quiz the students

C.  Use knowledge-based questioning with students
D.  Provide the students with an in-service training about critical thinking

*The correct answer is A. Role modeling is one of the most important aspects of teaching. In order for students to become professionals they must have professional role models.*

20. Which behavior by a student indicates that he or she has no knowledge deficit about basic safety standards?

A.  She introduces herself by first and last name to all of her patients.
B.  She refers to the patients by their room numbers.
C.  She asks the patients their names before dispensing medication.
D.  She discusses patients' conditions in the elevator.

*The correct answer is C. All students need to be concerned about safety and should use two identifiers with each patient.*

21. One of the main goals of self-directed learning (SDL) for students is to

A.  Comprehend the material better
B.  Build confidence
C.  Understand the facilitation role
D.  Become nurse educators

*The correct answer is B. Building confidence in one's own learning abilities is a primary goal of SDL.*

22. A nurse educator assesses the written work of a millennial generation student and is surprised that, in the references, the student uses:

A.  Text books
B.  Internet sources
C.  An encyclopedia
D.  Articles

*The correct answer is C. Millennial generation students typically use the Web to find electronic sources and for referencing.*

23. Number five of Gagne's nine learning steps has to do with assisting students as they organize information to assimilate it into their long-term memories. Organization and executive functioning is referred to as

A.  Metacognition
B.  Critical thinking
C.  Deep learning
D.  Cognitivism

*The correct answer is A. Metacognition is a function of thinking things through and relating them to what one already knows. ("I know that I know . . .")*

24. Nurse educators are challenged to "unlearn" at times in order to

    A. Put themselves in the students' shoes
    B. Open their minds to new ideas
    C. Break the situation down to simplest terms
    D. Incorporate previous knowledge

    *The correct answer is B. Unlearning is a term coined in knowledge development to go into a situation without any preconceived ideas.*

25. Due to the current nurse educator shortage, the goal of nurse educators should be to

    A. Put more material online
    B. Have teaching assistants (TAs)
    C. Mentor young educators
    D. Decrease program sizes

    *The correct answer is C. Reinforcing the professional workforce should be a primary goal for dealing with the nursing shortage.*

26. Students in a health assessment class are assessed at the end of the course in the learning laboratory to determine if the course objectives have been met. The best method to assess their learning in the three domains of learning would be to have the students:

    A. Develop a case study with questions
    B. Perform a specific assessment technique on another student
    C. Maintain a portfolio of assessment activities throughout the semester
    D. Write a summative journal entry about their learning for the course

    *The correct answer is B. Performing an assessment reveals cognitive (organization and accuracy of the exam), psychomotor (the skill needed to perform the exam), and affective (interaction with "the patient") capabilities.*

27. A student complains to a professor that he feels his paper was unfairly graded when compared to other students' papers. The professor's best response to the student would be:

    A. "The papers were graded based on the grading rubric described in the syllabus. Please review the comments I made on your paper."
    B. "Please submit your concerns to me in writing and I will review your paper to see if the grade can be changed."
    C. "If you submit a short essay, I will give you extra credit for this assignment."
    D. "I will give you extended time to revise the paper and resubmit it to me to improve your grade."

    *The correct answer is A. Providing a rubric is a good way to decrease subjectivity in an evaluation.*

28. The nursing program is preparing for a site visit by the National League for Nursing Accrediting Commission (NLNAC) and is preparing a self-study report. The main purpose of the visit is to:

   A. Determine the extent to which the program has achieved its mission, goals, and outcomes
   B. Assess the needs of the program
   C. Measure the strengths and weaknesses of the program
   D. Identify the program's admission standards

   *The correct answer is A. The NLNAC is concerned with whether nursing schools and colleges are living up to their mission and achieving goals that will enhance the profession.*

29. Which of the following assessment measures best provides an ongoing, evidence-based framework for assessing a nursing program's outcomes?

   A. NCLEX-RN pass rates
   B. Employer satisfaction surveys
   C. Student exit interviews
   D. A program evaluation plan

   *The correct answer is D. A program evaluation plan gives an overview of many aspects of the program.*

30. An instructor is preparing a formative evaluation of clinical performance for a student. It should include which of the following?

   A. A judgment as to whether or not the criteria have been met for the clinical experience.
   B. Identification areas that need improvement in clinical performance to meet objectives.
   C. Give a grade of pass/fail for the clinical rotation.
   D. Review anecdotal notes throughout the semester

   *The correct answer is B. Formative evaluations are done to help the student as he or she works to achieve desired outcomes by the end of the course.*

31. Achievement tests should be constructed so that they measure a representative sample of the test items relevant to the instruction. This is best accomplished by:

   A. Using a variety of types of tests, such as multiple-choice or essay
   B. Referring to the outcomes defined in the program evaluation plan
   C. Constructing a table of specifications for the learning unit
   D. Observing performance skills in the learning lab

   *The correct answer is C. Constructing a test plan that includes the content areas and shows their correct proportions is correct.*

32. Which of the following statements most accurately reflects criterion-referenced tests?

    A. "The student ranked in the 70th percentile on the nurse entrance exam."
    B. "Ninety percent of the students will correctly assess cranial nerves during the simulation skills lab."
    C. "The student achieved a score of 1250 on the SAT exam."
    D. "The student's cumulative GPA in the nursing courses is 3.2."

    *The correct answer is B. This estimation is based on the criteria for the course and is not based on the mean of the group.*

33. Which of the following provides more reliable test scores?

    A. Longer tests (more test items)
    B. Group homogeneity
    C. Forty-five percent of students answer a question correctly
    D. Very difficult test items

    *The correct answer is A. More test questions will increase the overall reliability of the test.*

34. An item analysis report reveals that the KR20 is 0.15. An educator can interpret this to mean that:

    A. The test was very reliable.
    B. The test measured a single factor, as intended.
    C. No changes need to be made to the test.
    D. The test did not measure what was intended.

    *The correct answer is D. The reliability of the test is low; therefore, the test was not reliable.*

35. The Admission and Progression committee in the nursing program is revising the progression standards in order to improve program outcomes. Which of the following is *not* a criterion for progression in the nursing program?

    A. A minimum grade of 80% is required for nursing and science courses.
    B. Students may repeat a nursing course one time.
    C. Junior level status must be achieved before beginning the nursing program.
    D. Students must achieve the national standard average on the ATI test.

    *The correct answer is C. "Junior level status" is interpreted differently by different institutions and is reliant on non-nursing criteria.*

36. The laboratory instructor has been teaching material that is extraneous to the skills that the students need to master. What is an appropriate way to deal with this?

A. Tell the students to ignore the material that the laboratory instructor gives them.
B. Demand that the instructor be removed from your course.
C. Advise the students that it will not hurt them to learn some additional material.
D. Review the material that is pertinent to the students' success with the instructor every week.

*The correct answer is D. Making a teaching plan is one of the best ways to hone a faculty member's focus.*

37. The characteristics of simulation include which of the following?

A. Simulations can take many forms
B. Trainees are placed in simple situations
C. Simulations are completely like the "real thing"
D. Simulations are always interactive

*The correct answer is A. Simulation experiences have endless possibilities.*

38. A clinical instructor can find no patients in her unit that meet the learning objectives for the week. What strategy should she implement to ensure her students meet their learning needs?

A. Take them back to the college laboratory and role-play the care of the patients.
B. Send them to other units in the hospital to observe the care of the patients with the appropriate diagnoses.
C. Make assignments that will reinforce the previous week's learning needs.
D. Send them to the library with specific objectives that will reinforce the week's work.

*The correct answer is C. Reinforcing last week's skills will increase the students' confidence and skills until other experiences can be found.*

39. An attribute a clinical teacher should possess is:

A. Knowledge of the facility and keeping students challenged
B. Spontaneous pre and post conferences
C. The ability to maintain a strict adherence to the daily plan
D. A sense of what the staff would like the students to do each week

*The correct answer is A. It is imperative to know the system in which you are teaching in order to provide students with a good experience.*

40. When a student's actions or inactions jeopardize patient safety, the instructor should be prepared to:

A. Let the student work through problems him or herself.
B. Jump in to role model the appropriate behavior.

    C. Take the student aside and help him or her to reprioritize.
    D. Reassign the student to a different patient.

*The correct answer is B. The faculty is, at times, a safety net for learning when a student's behavior jeopardizes patient safety.*

41. When the clinical group is large and the acuity of the patients is high, the clinical instructor may consider:

    A. Making dual or triple assignments
    B. Sending some students to the library with case studies to solve
    C. Taking the students on nursing rounds
    D. Assigning a patient to herself to demonstrate complex care

*The correct answer is A. Decreasing the number of patients to oversee is the safest alternative.*

42. Before giving a test, the faculty should develop a test blueprint that includes the:

    A. Scoring key
    B. Content that will be tested
    C. Percentage weights of some areas
    D. Scoring procedure

*The correct answer is B. Providing students with the content to be tested will decrease their anxiety and also role model the traits of transparency and fairness.*

43. An essay test enables an instructor to:

    A. Cover limited areas of knowledge
    B. Score exams quickly
    C. Determine how students organize their thoughts
    D. Measure facts efficiently

*The correct answer is C. Essays are a great evaluation method for thought organization.*

44. The most efficient way to evaluate students in the clinical area is to:

    A. Develop an objective test for each week's work
    B. Develop a system of anecdotal notes that can be synthesized at a specified time during the semester
    C. Video tape each student weekly to ensure accurate evaluation
    D. Develop a skills checklist that will act as a teaching and evaluative tool.

*The correct answer is B. Anecdotal notes have been used for years to verify subjective evaluations of students' skills, behavior, and performance.*

45. When developing or changing the curriculum, a leader's most appropriate action is to:

   A. Hurry the faculty through the process so that they do not have time to resist too much.
   B. Inform each faculty member individually of the change so that they cannot resist as a group.
   C. Give individuals an opportunity to express their opinions and concerns.
   D. Give optimistic speculations about the viability of the new curriculum.

   *The correct answer is C. The curriculum must be owned by the faculty in order for it to be an accepted change that works well.*

46. Which of the following would be an example of the scholarship of discovery?

   A. A Grant aware in support of research
   B. Theoretical development
   C. Professional role modeling
   D. Mentoring junior colleagues

   *The correct answer is B. Theoretical development is the scholarship of discovery.*

47. The process of giving new meaning to isolated facts is which of the following?

   A. The scholarship of discovery
   B. The scholarship of teaching
   C. The scholarship of integration
   D. The scholarship of clinical practice

   *The correct answer is C. Giving new meaning to isolated facts is the scholarship of integration. It not only gives new meaning to isolated facts, but may involve making connections across disciplines.*

48. Here is a list of scores. Please calculate what grade the student will have
   Quizzes: 98, 93, 96 count for 30% of the grade
   Tests scores: 97, 90, 89 count for 50% of the grade
   Projects scores: 85 and 94 count for 20% of the grade
   What grade will you give the student if an A = 93–100, A– = 90–92, B+ = 86–89, and B = 80–85

   A. The student will receive an A
   B. The student will receive a A–
   C. The student will receive a B+
   D. Not enough information is present

   *The answer is B. The student will receive an A–. To get the answer to this question you must add the scores 98–92–96 = 287 divide them by 3 = 95.6.*

*Multiply that by .30 = 28.68. Then for the tests you must add 97 + 90 + 89 = 276 and divide that by 3 = 92. Multiply that by .50 which will give you 46. For the projects add 85 + 94 which equals 89.5. Multiply that by .2 which = 17.9. To get the weighted score then add 26.8 + 46 + 17.9 = 92.58. 92.58 is an A– so the student will receive that grade.*

49. Which of the following has competence as the method by which knowledge in the profession is advanced?

    A. Scholarship of teaching
    B. Scholarship of discovery
    C. Scholarship of nursing
    D. Scholarship of practice

    *The answer is D, scholarship of practice. Competence is a practice issue and may include the direct care giver, and educator, a consultant, or an administrator.*

50. Which of the following requires participation from 2 or more disciplines working together?

    A. The scholarship of integration
    B. The scholarship of practice
    C. The scholarship of discovery
    D. The scholarship of teaching

    *The answer is A, the scholarship of integration. Usually this involves the discipline of nursing and another discipline.*

51. Which of the following are considered educational records under FERPA?

    A. private notes of an individual staff or faculty
    B. Campus police records
    C. statistical data that contains no personally identifiable information about a student
    D. A students posted assignment on the discussion board during an on-line class.

    *The answer is D. This is considered class work and considered part of the educational record under FERPA*

52. Peer reviewed published books would be considered

    A. Scholarship of teaching
    B. Scholarship of discovery
    C. Scholarship of integration
    D. Scholarship of practice

    *The answer is C, scholarship of integration*

53. In the American Disabilities Act of 1990, who has the primary responsibility for identifying and documenting disability to obtain accommodations?
   A. The teacher
   B. The student/learner
   C. The schools academic resource center
   D. The school psychologist

   *The answer is B. The student or learner has the primary responsibility for identifying and documenting disability and requesting specific supports, services, or other accommodations needed.*

54. The item analysis revealed the following data for a multiple-choice question:

   | Point Biserial = 0.29 | Correct answer = B | | Total group = 41% | |
   | --- | --- | --- | --- | --- |
   | Distractor Analysis: | A | B | C | D |
   | Pt-Biser.: | −0.25 | 0.39 | −0.35 | 0.19 |
   | Frequency: | 41% | 41% | 12% | 6% |

   *Based on these statistics the professor should do which of the following when using this item on future exams:*

   A. Remove the question because less than 50% of students got it correct
   B. Keep it the way it is because it was discriminating
   C. Revise distractor B to assist the students to choose it.
   D. Revise distractors A and D because they are not discriminating

   *The correct answer is D. The faculty should revise the distractors A & D because they produced negative point bi-serials therefore higher-level students choose them.*

55. In a clinical nursing course, 50% of the grade must be in by midterm. The student has an average of 72.5 at midterm. There is a comprehensive exam worth 50% at the end of the semester. What is the least grade needed on that exam to accomplish a course grade of 76%?
   A. 76.5%
   B. 79.5%
   C. 81.5%
   D. 83.5%

   *The correct answer is B. 76.5%. The midterm grade of 72.5% divide by .5 for 50% = 36.25. Subtract 36.25 from 76% and the remainder is 39.75. A 39.75 which is 50% of the grade now needs to be doubled = 79.5%. Or 72.5 + 79.5 = 152 and divide by 2 = 76 average.*

# Answers to End-of-Chapter Practice Questions

## Chapter 2 Practice Questions

1. The nurse educator should expect to observe the following characteristics in the reticent student:

   B. Inability to contribute to a group project

   *Correct answer is B. A reticent student is introverted and has difficulty in group situations.*

2. Which type of post-lesson questions should the nurse educator expect to be asked by beginning students who are visual learners when reviewing information from a tape of heart sounds?

   A. Knowledge-based questions

   *The correct answer is A. Test questions should be leveled so that beginning students should be exposed to more knowledge-based questions; as they progress through the program, the application and comprehension level questions should make up a larger percentage of the test.*

3. When assessing the capabilities of a freshman student in the lab during a simulated experience, a nurse educator should expect the student to be at which level of Bloom's Taxonomy about basic cardiac function?

   A. Knowledge

   *The correct answer is A. This is the same rationale as Question 3. In the beginning of the curriculum, knowledge-based questions should comprise the majority of test and lab questions.*

4. Which finding should the nurse educator *least* expect when assessing the learning outcomes in the current curriculum?

   B. The process is prescribed

   *The correct answer is B. The process is less important than the outcome in today's philosophical realm.*

5. Which finding should a nurse educator expect when evaluating a new faculty member in the classroom?

   A. Mild speaking anxiety

*The correct answer is A. New faculty members often have mild speaking anxiety; this is expected, especially if someone is watching them.*

6. When a nurse educator suspects a student has a learning disability, he or she should:

   B. Refer the student to the learning center

   *The correct answer is B. The student should be referred to the learning center for evaluation before accommodations are made in the classroom or clinical area.*

7. A nurse educator uses a tool to assess a class of students to determine the group's most prominent learning style. To elicit the information effectively, he or she should:

   B. Provide students with time in class to complete the assessment

   *The correct answer is B. Time in class should be provided so that results are readily available and everyone has a chance to be evaluated.*

8. When interviewing for a job, a nurse educator is asked about her education philosophy and says that she is primarily concerned with equality in the classroom. This nurse educator most likely subscribes to the philosophy of

   B. Emancipatory education

   *The correct answer is B. Emancipatory education is concerned with oppression and freedom in the classroom and the faculty as learning in the process.*

9. At a faculty retreat a nurse educator is telling the group about her philosophy and says, "I believe in rewarding students for good behavior and doing well on tests." What philosophy is the educator a proponent of?

   D. Behaviorism

   *The correct answer is D. Behaviorism evaluates an observed behavior in order to determine if learning has taken place.*

10. Which statement by a student should alert a nurse educator to difficulty with the material?

    D. "I understand the material in class, but cannot pick the right test answer."

    *The correct answer is D. Being unable to choose the correct answer usually has to do with distinguishing priorities in the presented material. The faculty member may consider emphasizing the most important nursing intervention or best nursing diagnoses for the content being presented.*

## Chapter 3 Practice Questions

1. A nurse educator is designing a program to assist culturally diverse learners in your university's courses. Which of the following strategies would be most beneficial for the educator to include?

D. Developing a mentor program that pairs learners with a faculty member.

*Correct answer is D. Evidence shows that the direct mentoring of culturally diverse students increases the learner's outcomes.*

2. A nurse educator is teaching an online course about the concepts of nursing. One of the learners has posted an opinion to the discussion board that is negative about the profession of nursing. Other students in the class have posted comments in agreement with the first posting. What should the nurse educator teaching the course do?

B. Courteously question the student's first posting and open a dialogue about the topic

*The correct answer is B. Presenting the opposite side of the position in a non-threatening environment is the best way to guide learners through a reflective discussion.*

3. A nurse educator recognizes that a student who is a visual learner would prefer which of the following assignments:

C. Create a concept map using a computer

*The correct answer is C. Concept mapping is an excellent learning activity for visual learners.*

4. The best example of a service learning project would be

B. Participating in a teddy bear clinic for course credit

*The correct answer is B. Although all options given could be considered service learning—the teddy bear clinic is a direct involvement with the community.*

5. A student does poorly on an exam and then approaches the educator to share that they have attention deficit hyperactivity disorder (ADHD). The student asks the educator if, in the future, they may take tests in another room and be given more time. What would be the best response to the student by the educator?

B. "Do you have a note from the learning center verifying this disorder?"

*The correct answer is B. A student should provide appropriate documentation verifying his or her learning disability.*

6. A student made a medication error in the clinical area during the pediatric rotation. The nurse educator could best demonstrate "role modeling" of the nursing profession and good socialization skills by doing which of the following?

B. Take the student aside in a private area to review the error made, notify the appropriate individuals, and fill out an internal incident report.

*The correct answer is B. Hold the student accountable and responsible for the mistake by following through.*

7. Which of the following is an example of a uncivil behavior by a student in the classroom? (Choose all that apply.)

    A. Talking to another student while the instructor is lecturing

    D. Asking a question of a teacher and then arguing with him or her, saying that the response is inaccurate

*The correct answers are A and D. Answers B and C could be construed as uncivil if they were acts of cheating, but A and D are incidents of open incivility.*

8. Which of the following phases is described by a student who just passed her licensure examination, is off of orientation, and is in her third week of taking a solo patient assignment in the critical care unit? Suddenly, her patient deteriorates, so she asks a senior nurse for help. The senior nurse responds, "Why don't you go ask your preceptor, I am too busy."

    B. Shock or rejection

*The correct answer is B. This is an example of reality shock in nursing, and occurs once the honeymoon phase is over.*

9. A novice educator just attended a conference on utilizing technology in an online course. Soon, she will be teaching her first online course. Which of the following statements would indicate the novice educator's need for additional learning?

    A. "I am so confident, I am going to use all of these technologies learned and I won't need any more technological help, what a relief!"

*The correct answer is A. Overconfidence in the teaching role is a "red flag" when exhibited by a novice educator. All faculty are life-long learners.*

10. In understanding cultural diversity of students in the classroom. You wrote a test question in which the best answer was for the student to choose a clear liquid to give the patient. During the exam, a Chinese student with English as a second language approaches you to ask you what "Gatorade" is. An astute educator should do which of the following:

    C. Realize that not all cultures are familiar with American food and drink, such as Gatorade as a clear liquid

*The correct answer is C. Cultural sensitivity involves placing yourself in another's situation and realizing that what is common for one person may not be for another.*

## Chapter 4 Practice Questions

1. The Program Evaluation committee of the nursing program is reviewing the program evaluation data. The nursing program has established an 86% pass rate as the benchmark for graduates taking the NCLEX-RN exam for the

first time. This goal has not been met for the past three years. Which of the following recommendations would be a priority for the committee to make?

B.   Require a minimum GPA of 3.0 in all natural science and nursing courses.

*The correct answer is B. Studies show that grades in science courses are an indicator of NCLEX-RN success.*

2.  A clinical instructor is preparing to write the summative evaluation for the students in her clinical group. She believes in the Constructivist philosophy of evaluation. Therefore, when completing the evaluation she will do which of the following?

C.   Seek input from clinical staff regarding each student's clinical performance.

*The correct answer is C. Constructivists use reality to evaluate learning, and the clinical staff is part of the clinical reality for each student.*

3.  The nursing curriculum committee is revising the curriculum to be more congruent with changes in health care delivery. The most important consideration of the committee should be which of the following?

A.   Be sure the new curriculum is aligned with the mission and philosophy of the governing institution.

*The correct answer is A. The first step in any curriculum change should be its alignment with the governing body or larger institution.*

4.  A nurse educator is reviewing the item analysis on a course test for a multiple-choice question. The following statistics were calculated for this item:

| Point Biserial = −0.27 | Correct Answer = B | | Total Group = 88.24% | |
|---|---|---|---|---|
| Distractor Analysis: | A | B | C | D |
| Pt-Biserial: | 0.27 | −0.27 | 0.00 | 0.00 |
| Frequency: | 12% | 88% | 0% | 0% |

*The educator realizes the cause for this frequency distribution is:*

C.   Students who scored lower on the exam got the item correct.

*The correct answer is C. A negative point biserial indicates that the distractor did not differentiate between learners' abilities.*

5.  The following statistics were calculated on a multiple-choice question on an exam:

| Point Biserial = 0.61 | Correct Answer = C | | Total Group = 76.47% | |
|---|---|---|---|---|
| Distractor Analysis: | A | B | C | D |
| Pt-Biserial: | −0.59 | 0.00 | 0.61 | −0.24 |
| Frequency: | 6% | 0% | 88% | 6% |

*The reason for this frequency distribution is:*

D. *Students who scored higher on the exam got the item correct.*

*Correct answer is D. This question differentiated between the abilities of the learners for this evaluation.*

6. The item analysis revealed the following data for a multiple-choice question:

| Point Biserial = 0.19 | Correct Answer = D | | Total Group = 5.88% | |
|---|---|---|---|---|
| Distractor Analysis: | A | B | C | D |
| Pt-Biserial: | −0.25 | 0.39 | −0.35 | 0.19 |
| Frequency: | 41% | 41% | 12% | 6% |

*Based on these statistics, the professor should do which of the following when using this item on future exams:*

C. *Revise distractor B*

*The correct answer is C. The faculty should revise the distractor B because it is wrong but produced a higher point biserial than the correct answer, this indicates that it "fooled" some of the better learners of this content.*

7. An item analysis report for a multiple-choice exam revealed that the KR20 was 0.56. Based on this statistic, which of the following interpretations can be made regarding this exam?

A. The exam is reliable in measuring student knowledge of the material.

*The correct answer is A. The KR20 indicates that this is a reliable evaluation.*

8. A professor administered a multiple-choice exam and performed an item analysis, which revealed the following data:

| Point Biserial = 0.56 | Correct Answer = A | | Total Group = 52.94% | |
|---|---|---|---|---|
| Distractor Analysis: | A | B | C | D |
| Pt-Biserial: | 0.56 | −0.31 | −0.44 | 0.02 |
| Frequency: | 52% | 18% | 18% | 12% |

*The likely cause for this frequency distribution is:*

B. *Students who scored highest on the exam got the item correct.*

*The correct answer is B. This is a very discriminating question because the higher scorers for this evaluation were able to choose the correct answer.*

9. The following statistics were obtained in an item analysis for a multiple-choice exam:

| Point Biserial = 0.00 | Correct Answer = C | | Total Group = 100% | |
|---|---|---|---|---|
| Distractor Analysis: | A | B | C | D |
| Pt-Biserial: | 0.00 | 0.00 | 0.00 | 0.00 |
| Frequency: | 0% | 0% | 100% | 0% |

*What action should be taken based on this data?*

D.  *Rewrite all of the distractors.*

*The correct answer is D. This question was easy for all the students and the distractors should be revised in order to be discriminating.*

10. Which of the following activities would be the best strategy to engage the visual learner at the cognitive and affective levels?

C.  Developing a concept map

*The correct answer is C. Visual learners do well using concept mapping as opposed to audio (hearing) and writing (tactile) methods of learning.*

## Chapter 5 Practice Questions

1. Planning for curriculum development should include which activity?

B.  Collecting the demographic data of the community

*The correct answer is B. The community that is being served by the educational institution will impact the demographics of the students and the students' experiences.*

2. When choosing a leader for a curriculum revision, the faculty should consider which of the following first?

A.  The specific work involved

*The correct answer is A. Some faculty may be more suited than others, depending on the task being sought by the group.*

3. A faculty member insists that her favorite disease, juvenile thrombocytopenic purpera, be included in the pediatric syllabus despite her colleagues concerns. Which is the best strategy for the leader to take?

C.  Remind her of her responsibility to adhere to the curriculum plan

*The correct answer is C. The faculty must work as a team in order to contribute to a successful curriculum plan.*

4. When developing the curriculum, the faculty will look to which of the following for their reason of being?

C.  Institutional mission/philosophy

*The correct answer is C. The institution or governing body is the starting point for any curriculum design. If the curriculum is not coherent with the mission of the institution, it will not benefit the faculty or learners.*

5. A graduate of the program identifies nursing as assessing, planning, implementing, and evaluating the care of clients and families with various health care needs. He most likely comes from a program model that is known as

    A.  Curriculum model

*The correct answer is A. The curriculum model is the model that uses the nursing process as a foundational basis.*

6.  Which curriculum model would include a course titled "Nursing Care of Clients with Respiratory Problems Across the Life Span"?

    B.  Integrated model

*The correct answer is B. Integrated models do not use systems or processes; they rely on human developmental stages.*

7.  When considering level outcomes, the educator must ensure that they progress logically to eventually reflect the:

    B.  Outcomes of the program

*The correct answer is B. Level objectives should feed into the "larger umbrella" of program objectives for a logical educational flow.*

8.  A nurse should use which of the following teaching strategies to reach the higher levels of Bloom's Taxonomy?

    D.  Questioning

*The correct answer is D. Questioning, sometimes called Socratic questioning, can be an effective method for reaching higher levels of understanding if the questions are not just knowledge-based and if they elicit critical thinking in the learner.*

9.  The students in your clinical group have requested that you provide them with some additional materials that will help them study for their next examination. What independent strategy would be appropriate?

    C.  A game addressing the material

*The correct answer is C. Gaming is an excellent, active way to facilitate small group learning.*

10.  Which teaching strategy requires considerable student preparation?

    C.  Debate

*The correct answer is C. A debate is an excellent critical thinking strategy, but it requires preparation time for both the learners and the faculty.*

## Chapter 6 Practice Questions

1.  Scott (1996) states that the first step in evaluating effectiveness of an organization is:

    C.  Establish standards to use for comparison

*The correct answer is C. Without comparable evaluation standards, the fairness in evaluation would be jeopardized.*

2. An indicator for evaluating the organizational effectiveness of a school of nursing from a structural perspective includes:

    D.   Faculty characteristics and qualifications

*The correct answer is D. The faculty are part of the structure, so to speak, of a program. The NCLEX-RN success rate does tell organizational effectiveness because it is an outcome indicator.*

3. An indicator for evaluating the organizational effectiveness of a school of nursing from an outcome perspective includes:

    B.   Number of students passing the NCLEX-RN

*The correct answer is B. The NCLEX-RN success rate does reveal organizational effectiveness because it is an outcome indicator.*

4. An individual's perception of an organization's openness to creativity is influenced by the presence of interactional factors such as:

    A.   Intellectual orientation

*The correct answer is A. Intellectual orientation is, in effect, the way in which an organization encourages creative thinkers to take risks and develop new projects.*

5. An individual's willingness to initiate creative efforts is influenced by:

    B.   Organizational openness

*The correct answer is B. Organizational openness sets the stage for faculty to take risks in trying new ideas and programs.*

6. Lewin's change theory is characterized by the presence of:

    B.   Driving and restraining forces

*The correct answer is B. Driving and restraining forces in a person and organization are major variables in Lewin's change theory.*

7. The Theory of Reasoned Action is characterized by the presence of:

    C.   Intention to perform an action

*The correct answer is C. Intention to change is the variable that sets off the cycle of change in the Theory of Reasoned Action.*

8. Lippitt's Phases of Change theory is characterized by the presence of:

    A.   The motivation and capacity for change

*The correct answer is A. Lippitt's theory uses motivation and capacity to predict change in people.*

9. An example of a faculty activity that supports recognition for service learning activities is:

    C.   Involving faculty in opportunities for publication

*The correct answer is C. Disseminating information to the wider nursing community can be considered service learning.*

10. An example of an institutional activity that supports planning for service learning activities is:

    B. Form an advisory committee

    *The correct answer is B. An advisory committee can look at the needs of the community and participants in order to plan service learning to meet the needs.*

## Chapter 7 Practice Questions

1. An example of a Web 2.0 social networking site is

   D. Facebook

   *The correct answer is D. Facebook is a social networking Web site used by a great number of college-aged students.*

2. A standardized patient is a

   C. An actor who portrays a patient with a medical condition

   *The correct answer is C. A standardized patient is actually a live actor or actress who plays the same "role" for any number of students.*

3. Mentoring nursing faculty includes which of the following

   D. All of the above

   *The correct answer is D. All the above attributes mentioned are necessary in order to have an effective mentor/mentee relationship.*

4. A comprehensive academic nurse educator orientation should include

   D. All of the above

   *The correct answer is D. All of the above topics are important for an orientation program for novice nurse educators or educators entering a new system.*

5. Which of the following describes a learner-directed activity

   D. A learning activity where the learner takes the initiative

   *The correct answer is D. To be truly learner-directed, the learners must initiate the activity.*

6. The elements of lifelong learning for the nurse educator vary according to

   D. All of the above

   *The correct answer is D. All of the above variables play a role in the learning objectives of a faculty member.*

7. A Wiki is

  A.   A collection of Web pages that are editable by anyone

*The correct answer is A. A Wiki page may be community edited, which is a point to keep in mind when using the information or seeking out information whose accuracy is vital.*

8. The Technology Informatics Guiding Education Reform (TIGER) Initiative is

  C.   A consortium of more than 40 nursing professional organizations that "aims to enable practicing nurses and nursing students to fully engage in the unfolding digital era of health care."

*The correct answer is C. TIGER is a consortium.*

9. Feedback during the faculty evaluation process can come from which of the following

  D.   All of the above

*The correct answer is D. All of the above formats can provide valuable feedback for any faculty member.*

10. Mentoring is

  D.   All of the above

*The correct answer is D. Mentoring involves all of the above criteria and is a professional relationship that focuses on reciprocity.*

# Chapter 8 Practice Questions

1. A nurse educator is preparing a dossier for promotion to Associate Professor. The university uses Boyer's Model of Scholarship to guide the development of the dossier. The nurse educator is providing evidence for the scholarship of application. The nurse educator should include which of the following examples to demonstrate excellence in the scholarship of application?

  B.   Service on a task force of a national nursing organization in which the educator shares expertise about use of rubrics in evaluating learning outcomes.

*The correct answer is B. Application is using one's knowledge to assist the community in solving issues concerning education.*

2. The curriculum committee at a school of nursing is debating the best way to sequence clinical learning experiences. The committee should first

  C.   Review the published evidence.

*The correct answer is C. Evidence-based education should guide the decisions of a program to ensure the best outcome.*

3. A nurse educator uses concept maps for the first time with nursing students in an accelerated program. The nurse educator is demonstrating which of the following?

   A. Good teaching

   *The correct answer is A. This is an activity that demonstrates good teaching because it is evidence-based education. Concept mapping has been demonstrated to increase learners' critical thinking.*

4. A nurse educator has completed a funded study about the effectiveness of the use of Podcasts for nursing students with learning styles preferences for auditory learning. Which of the following is the most effective way to share results of this study?

   A. Publish in a nursing education journal.

   *The correct answer is A. Disseminating information to the wider nursing community is the best way to let others know about a teaching strategy that produced desired outcomes.*

5. Which of the following is the most effective form of peer review for scholarly work?

   D. Grant funding from an agency external to the campus

   *The correct answer is D. Grant fundings are peer reviewed proposals that are usually competitive and, therefore, well scrutinized.*

6. A nurse educator wants to determine the effectiveness of using "debriefing" after a simulation in which students in her classroom interpreted an EKG and selected interventions for a critically ill "patient." In order to obtain funding for this study, the nurse educator should first submit a proposal to

   B. Campus small grants program for teaching innovations

   *The correct answer is B. Internal grants are a great mechanism for funding small or pilot programs.*

   [Brenda Reap-Thomson contributed the following questions.]

7. The nurse educator analyzed data and reported outcomes of the safety regulations in an outpatient center. This would be an example of:

   D. Scholarship of practice (application)

   *The correct answer is D. The Scholarship of practice includes activities that have a direct impact on clients' health care.*

8. The students are encouraged to become members of the National Student Nurses' Association. The framework for this organization indicates that the students will gain experience:

   A. Making decisions and being held accountable for those decisions.

*The correct answer is A. The framework for this organization is shared governance, therefore students will have the opportunity to discuss their opinions and make decisions. The group members are responsible for the outcome of decisions.*

9. The university has received a grant to support the remedial education of minority students; this will provide assistance for more minorities' entrance into nursing. This would be an example of:

   D.  Program grants

   *The correct answer is D. Program grants support target groups.*

   A.  *Research grants are used for the study of a specific concept.*
   B.  *Scholarship grants are used to finance the cost of education.*
   C.  *Training grants are used for professional development.*

10. A nurse educator is applying for a promotion. It would be of greatest advantage to

    A.  Write an article in a refereed journal

    *The correct answer is A. Refereed journals are peer reviewed and are considered to carry a greater degree of credibility and prestige.*

# Chapter 9 Practice Questions

*Contributed by Brenda Reap-Thompson.*

1. The nurse educator is discussing graduation with students. One of the students says that being responsible for clients without the presence of an instructor is very frightening. Which statement by the nurse educator would be most appropriate?

   D.  "Your mentor will provide a structured process to guide your decisions and behaviors."

   *The correct answer is D. The mentor, working along side the student, provides guidance during everyday client care, decision-making, and teaching.*

2. The school of nursing has implemented a standardized examination to be administered at the mid-curriculum completion point. What is the purpose of the examination? Select all that apply

   A.  Identify students who are below the benchmark.
   B.  Determine if there is a need to revise the curriculum.
   C.  Provide another method of testing to add to the student grade.
   D.  Collect data which can be u sed for informational purposes.

   *The correct answers are A, B, C, and D. The mid-curriculum examination may be initiated for multiple reasons. It is commonly used to identify students who are at risk for failure of NCLEX-RN. The results can be used to determine areas for remediation in order to progress.*

3. A nurse educator is mentoring a new educator. The new educator looks stressed and says, "I had some problems with the class, but I know things will get better." Which of the following responses would be appropriate?

A. "Tell me about your class."

*The correct answer is A. This is an open-ended question that will progress to a conversation.*

4. A nurse educator is teaching a large class that is very diverse. Which population of students is at increased risk for failure?

C. Students who speak English as a Second Language (ESL)

*The correct answer is C. Students who speak English as a Second Language (ESL) are at increased risk of being unsuccessful in the program and on the NCLEX-RN.*

5. A nurse educator has a student in class who receives accommodations for increased time for testing because of a disability. The faculty needs to:

C. Accommodate the student.

*The correct answer is C. Faculty need to accommodate the student as indicated.*

6. A student who was unsuccessful in the course tells a faculty member that she does not think it was her fault she failed. She said that she came to every class, but that the tests were unfair. Which of the following statements by the faculty would be appropriate?

A. "You can appeal the grade if you think it was unfair."

*The correct answer is A. Students have the right to appeal a grade if they believe it was unfair. There are specific guidelines that can be found in the student handbook.*

7. The chair of the Curriculum Committee is known as a transformational leader. This indicates that the leader:

D. Energized the committee to perform at a high level.

*The correct answer is D. A transformational leader encourages the group and fosters enthusiasm, which results in high quality work with increased productivity.*

8. A clinical instructor provided learning opportunities for four students. Which of the following clinical experiences reflects use of the affective domain?

C. Interviewing a client who was diagnosed last week with breast cancer.

*The correct answer is C. The affective domain means learning is in a social context. Observing a nurse discuss issues with a family member or watching a video about death and dying are also examples.*

9. A faculty member is completing a peer review. During the adult health class, the students sit quietly; some learners take notes, and some just listen to the lecture. Which of the following information would be appropriate to suggest?

   B. Initiate a game that involves all students for a quick review of content.

   *The correct answer is B. Games, such as Jeopardy, bingo, or responding to a question when one catches a ball are all active learning techniques that engage students and increase their understanding of concepts. Choices A, C, and D do not promote active learning.*

10. The course data demonstrates that 97% of the class passed the course. The class average on the customized specialty external examination, which is 15% of the grade, was 70.5%. Which conclusion can be drawn from this data?

    A. The internal curriculum evaluation should be reviewed.

    *The correct answer is A. The internal curriculum, which is the measurement of student outcomes according to course objectives such as examinations, quizzes, presentations and research papers, should be reviewed for rigor. The students did poorly on the external examination (HESI, ATI), which is a standardized test. The external examination is significant because it compares students to a larger population of learners.*

11. A nurse educator taught cardiac rhythms, code management and medications in the Adult Critical Care Course. What would be the *most* effective method of determining the students' understanding of the information?

    C. Schedule a simulation experience that will encompass the chapter objectives.

    *The correct answer is C. Simulation will provide students with the experience without placing any clients at risk. It will also give the students immediate feedback if they administered an incorrect medication or completed an incorrect intervention.*

# Additional Study Resources

## Highly Recommended

Billings, D. M., & Halstead, J. A. (2009). *Teaching in nursing: A guide for faculty* (3rd ed.). St. Louis, MO: Elsevier Saunders.

Gaberson, K. B., & Oermann, M. H. (2006). *Clinical teaching strategies in nursing.* New York: Springer Publishing.

Moyer, B. A., & Wittmann-Price, R. A. (2008). *Nursing education: foundations for practice excellence.* Philadelphia: F.A. Davis Company.

Novotny, J. M., & Quinn-Griffin, M. T. (2006). *A nuts-and-bolts approach to teaching nursing* (3rd ed.). New York: Springer Publishing.

Oermann, M. H., & Gaberson, K. B. (2009). *Evaluation and testing in nursing education* (3rd ed). New York: Springer Publishing.

## Recommended

Angelo, T., & Cross, K. P. (1993). *Classroom assessment techniques: A handbook for college teachers* (2nd ed.). San Francisco: Jossey-Bass.

Bastable, S. B. (2008). *Nurse as educator: Principles of teaching and learning for nursing practice* (3rd ed.). Sudbury, MA: Jones and Bartlett Publishers.

Bates, A. W., & Poole, G. (2003). *Effective teaching with technology in higher education: Foundations for success.* San Francisco: Jossey-Bass.

Bevis, E. O., & Watson, J. (2000). *Toward a caring curriculum: A new pedagogy for nursing.* Sudbury, MA: Jones and Bartlett Publishers.

Boyer, E. (1990). *Scholarship reconsidered: Priorities of the professoriate.* Princeton, NJ: The Carnegie Foundation for the Advancement of Teaching.

Caputi, L., & Engelmann, L. (2004). *Teaching nursing: The art and science* (Vols. 1, 2, & 3). Glen Ellyn, IL: College of DuPage Press.

Clark, C. C. (2008). *Classroom skills for nurse educator.* Boston: Jones and Bartlett Publishers.

Cross, P. K. (1996). *Classroom Research: Implementing the scholarship of teaching.* San Francisco: Jossey-Bass.

DeYoung, S. (2009). *Teaching strategies for nurse educators.* Upper Saddle River, NJ: Prentice Hall.

Dick, W., Carey, L., & Carey, J. (2005). *The systematic design of instruction* (6th ed.). New York: Pearson Education.

Diekelmann, N. L. (Ed.). (2003). *Teaching the practitioners of care: New pedagogies for the health professions.* Madison, WI: The University of Wisconsin Press.

Drago-Severson, E. (2004). *Becoming adult learners: principles and practices for effective development.* New York: Teacher's College Press.

Dunn, R., & Griggs, S. A. (1998). *Learning styles and the nursing profession.* New York: Jones and Bartlett Publishers.

Ferguson, V. D. (Ed.). (1997). *Educating the 21st century nurse: Challenges & opportunities.* New York: NLN Press.

Gronlund, N. E. (2004). *Writing instructional objectives for teaching and assessment* (7th ed.). Upper Saddle River, NJ: Pearson/Merrill Prentice Hall.

Grossman, S., & Valiga, T. (2005). *The new leadership challenge: Creating the future of nursing.* Philadelphia: F.A. Davis Company.

Hannah, K. J., Ball, M. J., & Edwards, M. J. A. (2006). *Introduction to nursing informatics* (3rd ed.). New York: Springer Publishing.

Iwasiw, C. L., Goldenberg, D., & Andrusyszyn, M. (2009). *Curriculum development in nursing education* (2nd ed.). Boston: Jones and Bartlett Publishers.

Jackson, M., Ignatavicius, D., & Case, B. (2006). *Thinking and clinical judgment.* Boston Jones and Bartlett Publishers.

Keating, S. (2005). *Curriculum development and evaluation in nursing.* Philadelphia: Lippincott, Williams and Wilkins.

Kelly, M. L., & Fitzsimmons, V. M. (2000). *Understanding cultural diversity: Culture, curriculum, and community in nursing.* Sudbury, MA: Jones and Bartlett Publishers.

Knowles, M., Holton, E., & Swanson, R. (2005). *The adult learner: The definitive classic in adult education and human resource development* (6th ed.). St. Louis, MO, Elsevier.

Lawler, P., & King, P. (2000). *Planning for effective faculty development: using adult learning strategies.* Malabar, FL: Krieger Publishing Company.

McDonald, M. E. (2002). *Systematic assessment of learning outcomes: Developing multiple-choice exams.* Sudbury, MA: Jones and Bartlett Publishers.

McDonald, M. E. (2008). *The nurse educator's guide to assessing learning outcomes.* (2nd ed.). Boston: Jones and Bartlett Publishers.

McKeachie, W. J. (2002). *Teaching tips: Strategies, research and theory for college and university teachers* (11th ed.). New York: Houghton Mifflin Co.

O'Connor, A. B. (2006). *Clinical instruction and evaluation: A teaching resource.* Sudbury, MA: Jones and Bartlett Publishers.

Palloff, R. M., & Pratt, K. (2003). *The virtual student: A profile and guide to working with online learners.* San Francisco: Jossey-Bass.

Palmer, P. (1998). *The courage to teach: A guide for reflection and renewal.* San Francisco: Jossey-Bass.

Porter-O'Grady, T., & Malloch, K. (2003). *Quantum leadership: A textbook of new leadership.* Sudbury, MA: Jones and Bartlett Publishers.

Richardson, V. (2001). *Handbook of Research on Teaching* (4th ed.). Washington, DC: American Educational Research Association.

Wlodkowski, R. J., & Ginsberg, M. B. (2003). *Diversity & motivation: Culturally responsive teaching.* San Francisco: Jossey-Bass.

Wergin, J. (2003). *Departments that work: Building and sustaining cultures of excellence in academic programs.* Boston: Anker Publishing Co.

## Suggested Journals

*Assessment and Evaluation in Higher Education*
*EduCause Review*
*Higher Education Research and Development*
*International Journal of Nursing Education Scholarship*
*Journal of Continuing Education in Nursing*
*Journal of Nursing Education*
*Journal of Professional Nursing*
*Nurse Education in Practice*
*Nurse Education Today*
*Nursing Education Perspectives*
*Nurse Educator*
*Quality in Higher Education*
*Teachers and Teaching: Theory and Practice*
*Teaching and Higher Education*

## Related Web Sites

Agency for Healthcare Research and Quality. (2008). *Evidence Based Practice Centers.* Retrieved December 30, 2008, from http://www.ahrq.gov/clinic/epc/

Bond, L. (1996). *Norm and Criterion Referenced Testing.* Retrieved December 30, 2008, from http://pareonline.net/getvn.asp?v=5&n=2

Bressoud, D. (n.d.). *The One-minute paper.* Retrieved December 30, 2008, from http://www.maa.org/SAUM/maanotes49/87.html

Brown, B. (n.d.). *New Learning Strategies for Generation X*. Retrieved December 30, 2008, from http://www.ericdigests.org/1998–1/x.htm

Clark, D. M. (2007). *Learning Domains or Bloom's Taxonomy*. Retrieved December 30, 2008, from http://www.nwlink.com/~Donclark/hrd/bloom.html

Cooperative Learning. (n.d.). Retrieved December 30, 2008, from http://edtech.kennesaw.edu/intech/cooperativelearning.htm

Driscoll, M. O. (2002). How People Learn (and what technology might have to do with it). Retrieved December 30, 2008, from http://www.ericdigests.org/2003–3/learn.htm

*Evidence Based Practice.* (n.d.). Retrieved December 30, 2008, from http://www.biomed.lib.umn.edu/learn/ebp/#

*Evidence Based Nursing Education.* (2008). Retrieved December 30, 2008, from https://www.ncsbn.org/350.htm

Fleming, N. (2008). A Guide to Learning *Styles*. Retrieved December 30, 2008, from http://www.vark-learn.com/english/index.asp

Forehand, M. (2008). Bloom's Taxonomy. Retrieved December 30, 2008, from http://projects.coe.uga.edu/epltt/index.php?title=Bloom%27s_Taxonomy

Lieb, S. (n.d.). *Principles of Adult Learning*. Retrieved December 30, 2008, from http://honolulu.hawaii.edu/intranet/committees/FacDevCom/guidebk/teachtip/adu lts-2.htm

National League of Nursing. (2007). *Mentoring of Nursing Faculty Toolkit*. Retrieved December 30, 2008, from http://www.nln.org/facultydevelopment/mentoringToolkit/index.htm

Parude, K., & Morgan, P. (2008). Millennials Considered: A New generation, New Approaches, and Implications for Nursing Education. *Nursing Education Perspectives, 29*(2), 74–79. Retrieved May 1, 2009, from http://nln.allenpress.com/nlnonline/?request=get-document&issn=1536–5026&volume=029&issue=02&page=0074

*Problem Based Learning Online Resources.* (2002). Retrieved December 30, 2008, from http://pbl.cqu.edu.au/content/online_resources.htm

*Putting video lectures on the Web.* (n.d.). Retrieved December 30, 2008, from http://www.ilrt.bris.ac.uk/bblt/video.html

*What's your learning style?* (n.d.). Retrieved December 30, 2008, from http://www.usd.edu/trio/tut/ts/style.html

# Index